Implant Dental Nursing

This book is dedicated to past, present and future dental nurses

Implant Dental Nursing

Edited by

Mary Miller

RDN, MA in Education and Professional Studies, FHEA
Principal, Education and Training (Accredited)
Assessment Centre for Dental Nurses

Eastman Dental Hospital, London

Membership of Organisations

General Dental Council
British Association of Dental Nurses
National Examining Board for Dental Nurses
Higher Education Academy

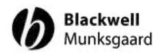
Blackwell
Munksgaard

Blackwell Munksgaard, a Blackwell Publishing Company,
Blackwell Publishing Ltd, 9600 Garsington Road, Oxford OX4 2DQ, UK
Tel: +44 (0)1865 776868
Blackwell Publishing Professional, 2121 State Avenue, Ames, Iowa 50014-8300, USA
Tel: +1 515 292 0140
Blackwell Publishing Asia Pty Ltd, 550 Swanston Street, Carlton, Victoria 3053, Australia
Tel: +61 (0)3 8359 1011

First published 2008 by Blackwell Munksgaard Ltd

ISBN: 978-1-4051-4428-5

Library of Congress Cataloging-in-Publication Data

Implant dental nursing / edited by Mary Miller.
p. ; cm.
Includes bibliographical references and index.
ISBN-13: 978-1-4051-4428-5 (pbk. : alk. paper)
ISBN-10: 1-4051-4428-9 (pbk. : alk. paper)   1. Dental implants.   2. Dental assistants.   I. Miller, Mary, 1951–
[DNLM: 1. Dental Implantation–methods.   2. Dental Implantation–nursing. 3. Dental Implants.   WU 640 I32 2008]

RK667.I45I42 2008
617.6′92–dc22
2007018850
A catalogue record for this title is available from the British Library

Set in 10 on 12 pt Sabon by SNP Best-set Typesetter Ltd., Hong Kong

The publisher's policy is to use permanent paper from mills that operate a sustainable forestry policy, and which has been manufactured from pulp processed using acid-free and elementary chlorine-free practices. Furthermore, the publisher ensures that the text paper and cover board used have met acceptable environmental accreditation standards.

For further information on Blackwell Munksgaard, visit our website:
www.dentistry.blackwellmunksgaard.com

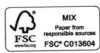

Contents

Authors

Ulpee R Darbar, BDS, FDSRCS, MSc, FDS (Rest Dent), RCS, ILTM
Consultant in Restorative Dentistry
Department of Restorative Dentistry
Eastman Dental Hospital
265 Gray's Inn Road
London WC1X 8LD

email: u.darbar@eastman.ucl.ac.uk

Membership of Organisations
General Dental Council (Registration No. 61207)
Medical Defence Union (Membership No. 2055751)
British Dental Association (Membership No. 0612079)

Suzanne Morkus, RDN, CERT Ed, Dip DH Ed
Tutor Dental Nurse
Education and Training (Accredited) Assessment Centre for Dental Nurses
Eastman Dental Hospital
265 Gray's Inn Road
London WC1X 8LD

email: suzanne.morkus@uclh.nhs.uk

Membership of Organisations
National Examining Board for Dental Nurses

Preface

Continual professional development is imperative for all members of the dental team, especially now for dental nurses since statutory registration with the General Dental Council in July 2007. This textbook is written to encourage dental nurses in their continual quest to enhance their knowledge and skills so that they can continue to be effective members of the dental team.

Dental implants are becoming more and more commonplace as patients expect to be offered them as part of a treatment plan. This textbook may be used as a guide when first encountering implants in the dental surgery or as an *aide memoire*, and will be useful to all members of the dental team.

Acknowledgements

My grateful thanks to Ulpee R Darbar and Suzanne Morkus, who found time in their busy schedules to write the chapters. Also to Rabiah Hussain for typing the manuscript.

History of dental implants

Dental implants have changed prosthetic reconstruction in the twenty-first century and opened doors to many patients who were once defined as dental cripples. The introduction of successful implant systems has meant that patients who have lost their own teeth have the opportunity to have replacement teeth like their own, thus maintaining their quality of life. Today what was once deemed an experimental treatment has now become the standard of care for patients with missing teeth. The advances in the field of implants have been reflected in the steady demand for and growth of dentistry in this area.

A dental implant is a device placed within, or on, the bone of the jaw (maxilla or mandible) to provide support for a prosthetic reconstruction, which could be a single tooth, multiple teeth or all the teeth, for example a denture. The use of such devices to replace lost teeth dates back to ancient times, and archeological findings have shown that ancient Egyptian and South American civilizations experimented with re-implanting lost teeth with hand-shaped ivory or wood substitutes.

In the eighteenth century attempts were made to use extracted teeth from human donors to replace missing teeth. The success rate was poor because of rejection by the recipient of the implanted teeth. Other attempts at using gold implants placed into fresh extraction sockets were reported in 1887. The first report by a physician using a platinum post for the same purpose was made in the late 1880s. Since this time implantation attempts using different metal alloys and porcelains have been reported with poor success rates because of rejection by body tissues.

In 1937 Strock reported on the first series of vitallium (an alloy of cobalt, chromium and molybdenum) implants placed into extraction sockets in animals and humans with no untoward postoperative complications or reactions. Histological specimens taken from the animals showed a good tissue tolerance to these implants, and follow-up of up to 15 years has shown the successful use of these implants to replace missing teeth. Since this time various other implant concepts and implants have been developed and these form the basis of modern-day implantology. Dental implants used today vary in several aspects, such as shape, place of anchorage (within or on the top of the bone), and the coating and composition of the material from which they are made. They can be categorized into three groups:

- subperiosteal implants
- transosseous implants
- endoosseous implants.

Subperiosteal implants

Subperiosteal implants lie on top of the jaw bone but underneath the gingival tissue, and they do not penetrate the jaw bone. These implants are mainly used for severely resorbed jaw bones where there is inadequate bone height, compromising the denture-bearing area and thus affecting the retention of the dentures. This type of implant has been in use successfully for the past 30 years and has the longest period of clinical use of any implant; the concept of which has been around for 60 years. The first subperiosteal implant was placed in 1948 by Gustav Dahl. The implant is shaped to rest on the residual bone ridge of either the maxilla or mandible, but is most commonly used in the mandible. The implant is custom made to each individual jaw and is made of a metal framework, shaped according to the jaw anatomy and surgically inserted underneath the periosteum. On completion of the surgery the metal inserts or bar (depending on the design used) visibly project from the gingival tissue. The denture carries an internal attachment which clips onto the projecting inserts, thus aiding retention. The denture is commonly made within 2–3 weeks of the implant being inserted (see Figs 1.1a, b, c).

Since the original implant, the design of the superiosteal implant has changed significantly in an attempt to improve success rates. Although long-term data reporting the success of these implants have been documented, the most common complication is fracture of the framework and resulting infection.

Transosseous implants

These implants are designed mainly for use in the mandible and are surgically inserted into the jaw bone; however, they penetrate through the entire jaw so that they emerge opposite the entry site, most commonly through the jaw at the

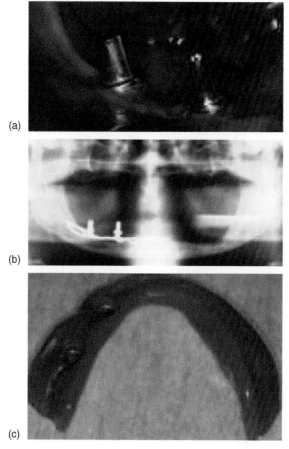

Figure 1.1 **(a)** Clinical picture of a subperiosteal implant. The prongs projecting into the mouth will retain the denture. **(b)** Radiograph showing the subperiosteal framework sitting on the alveolar bone. **(c)** The fitting surface of the denture showing the metal inserts which fit into the projecting prongs in the mouth

bottom of the chin. At this site they are secured with a pressure plate and nut. Two long screws penetrate the jaw bone and emerge from the gingival tissue. Separate attachments are placed on the screws projecting from the gingivae onto which the prosthesis is retained (see Fig. 1.2).

These implants require an extra-oral surgical approach and often necessitate the use of general anaesthesia. They are a type of endoosseous implant as they are screwed through the jaw bone. The success rates of these implants have remained questionable. This, in conjunction with the complexity of the procedure, has resulted in the demise of these implants, especially as other endoosseous implants are much more reliable.

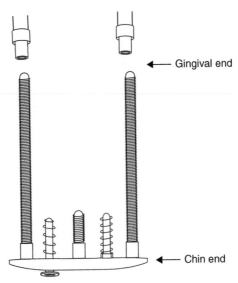

Figure 1.2 Transosseous implant. The plate at the bottom of the picture sits on the lower border of the jaw bone in the chin area. The two long screws penetrate the height of the jaw bone and emerge from the gingival tissue. Attachments on these two projections help to retain the denture

Endoosseous implants

These implants are surgically inserted into the jaw bone and can be grouped into three categories:

- ramus implants
- blade implants
- osseointegrated implants.

The Ramus implant

This implant is designed for the severely resorbed edentulous mandible. The resorption needs to be even. The implant comes in a standard preformed frame and has to be customized to fit the patient's jaw bone. It is surgically inserted and fixed to the bone in three areas: the chin area at the front of the mouth and the right and left back areas (around the last molar teeth). The implant is allowed to integrate with the jaw bone for 3 months. In a similar way to the subperiosteal implant, a bar projects above the gingival tissue into which the implant is inserted. This tripod stabilization offers advantages with improved stability but also reduces the risk of fracture in these very thin mandibles (see Figs 1.3a, b).

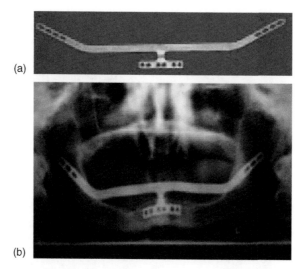

Figure 1.3   (a) A Ramus frame implant. (b) The Ramus frame implant in situ

Blade implants

These implants are also known as endosteal blade implants. They were first introduced by Linkow in the late 1960s. Their name is derived from the flat blade-like portion of the implant, which is the part that is embedded into the jaw bone (see Figs 1.4a, b). Although they have a long track record, there are hardly any documented reports. These implants are not commonly used today because of problems with failure related to infection and soft tissue damage. Their indication for use was in areas with compromised bone, but today they have been largely superseded by osseointegrated implants. It has been postulated that these implants function by developing a pseudoligament, but it is more likely that there is a soft tissue interface between the implant and the bone, which contributes to the loss of bony support and the development soft tissue infection, which is seen with time.

Osseointegrated implants

The second generation of dental implants is the osseointegrated dental implants. Their success has changed the philosophy surrounding the replacement of missing teeth. The concept was originally introduced by a Swedish research team headed by Per Ingvar Brånemark, an orthopaedic surgeon, in 1952. They studied microscopic bone-healing events in rabbits and found after several months of healing that the titanium metal cylinder in the implant had fused to the bone. Brånemark called this phenomenon osseointegration and proceeded, with a team from other disciplines, to research the use of titanium appliances in human bone, including the use of titanium screws as bone anchors for teeth. In the 1960s the

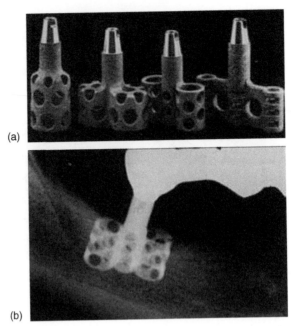

(a)

(b)

Figure 1.4   **(a)** The blade vent implants. **(b)** A radiograph showing a single tooth retained on a blade implant

development of a novel implant designed as a cylindrical titanium screw with a specific surface treatment to enhance its bioacceptance was tested. This screw depended on direct bone anchorage for clinical function and whilst it was believed that the oral implant was embedded in soft tissues, animal experiments undertaken at the Brånemark laboratory indicated that direct bone anchorage of the implant was possible provided that a number of guidelines were closely followed (details of these are provided in Chapter 2). Despite the successful outcome of this type of screw in human trials, it wasn't until 1981, when a landmark paper was published on this concept and subsequently presented at the Toronto Conference in 1982, that the concept of osseointegration became a worldwide accepted phenomenon. Figs 1.5a and b show a patient rehabilitated with osseointegrated implants.

Since the early 1980s the concept of osseointegrated implants has undergone tremendous development, with different materials, including aluminium oxide, commercially pure titanium and titanium alloys, being used for the implants. Additionally, surface coatings and surface alterations to improve integration alongside different shapes of implants have been introduced to enhance the integration rate to the jaw bone.

Endosseous osseointegrated implants have today become the norm for the replacement of missing teeth. There are currently in excess of 250 implant systems on the market based on the concept of osseointegration, reporting high success rates over 3–20 years. Many are replicas of the Brånemark system, but

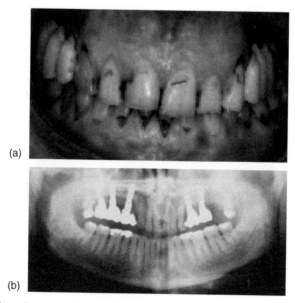

(a)

(b)

Figure 1.5   (a) Clinical picture and (b) radiograph showing a patient rehabilitated with endoosseous-osseointegrated implants

others with different designs have been developed. The basic concept and philosophy, however, remain the same.

Implant restorations

An implant-retained construction is made up of two parts. The part that is surgically placed is called the implant or fixture, whereas the actual tooth or teeth that go on top of the implant are called the prostheses. Osseointegrated implants are also called root form implants because they resemble the shape of the original root of the lost tooth. The events leading to the use of these implants to replace missing teeth can generally be divided into two phases, which are covered in detail in later chapters:

- the surgical phase involves all the procedures that are necessary to place the implant into the jaw bone to facilitate the prosthetic phase
- the prosthetic phase includes everything required to put a tooth or teeth on top of the implant(s).

Following the surgical phase the implant is allowed to integrate with the jaw bone for a period of up to 6 months; however, with advancing technology and different implant surfaces, this time has been reduced to 8 weeks or less. Once integrated the implant is then ready for the prosthetic phase, in which the prosthesis is constructed. The prosthesis can be either fixed to the implants or removable. The latter type can be removed by the patient for cleaning.

Factors affecting osseointegration

2

Osseointegrated implants, devices that are screwed or tapped into the alveolar and/or basal bone of the mandible or maxilla to support a prosthesis, have revolutionized the replacement of missing teeth with success rates of 85–95% both for edentulous (all teeth are missing) and partially dentate (some teeth or a single tooth are missing) patients. Once screwed into position the bone grows into the threads and crevices of the screw, thus anchoring it firmly into position to resemble a tooth root (see Fig. 2.1).

Although the development of the osseointegrated implants is attributed originally to the work of Brånemark and his co-workers in the late 1960s, Schroder and his team in the late 1970s, through a different series of experiments with histological data, reported the same findings (see Fig. 2.2). Both teams had shown through a series of experiments that direct bone anchorage exists between titanium and bone. They called this phenomenon osseointegration (see Fig 2.3).

Osseointegration was originally defined on a histological basis as a direct structural and functional connection between ordered and living bone, and the surface of a load-carrying implant (Brånemark et al. 1969). However, as the phenomenon of osseointegration became better understood, it was noted that 100% bone connection to the implant does not occur. Zarb and Albrektsson (1991) thus redefined osseointegration based on the clinical parameter of stability as 'a process whereby clinically asymptomatic and rigid fixation of an alloplastic material is achieved, and maintained, in bone during functional loading'. Once established, the osseointegrated interface of the bone to implant is relatively resistant to breaking down, although continuous exposure to adverse conditions, such as continuous overload, can lead to the breakdown of this

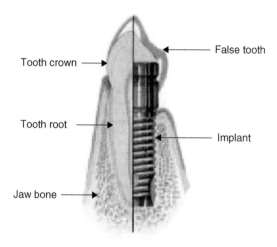

Tooth crown ——→

False tooth ←———

Tooth root ——→

Implant ←———

Jaw bone ——→

Figure 2.1   The comparison of an implant-retained crown with that of a tooth

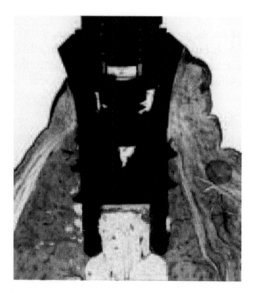

Figure 2.2   Histological section showing bone formation around an implant

interface causing implant failure and subsequently loss of the implant. Osseo-integration has been shown to be a time-related phenomenon and is dependent on the environment the implant is placed in as well as the surface finish of the implant. When originally developed, the earlier endoosseous implants needed up to 6 months for osseointegration to occur; however, today shorter time frames ranging from 1 to 3 months have been reported with some implant systems. The latter is associated with an implant surface that encourages the bone cells

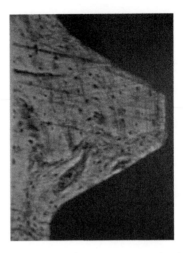

Figure 2.3   Section showing the bone to implant contact around a titanium surface

to be attracted to the implant surface at a faster rate, thus encouraging osseointegration to occur much faster than originally postulated.

A number of other factors can also influence the ability of the implant to osseointegrate successfully into the jaw bone. These can be divided into two categories:

- those that are related to the implant itself
- those that relate to the host bed and the bone into which the implant is going to be placed.

In addition to these categories, patient-related factors, which often have an effect on the host bed, may also influence the outcome and success. These are covered in Chapter 6.

Factors relating to the implant

Biocompatibility

The material of which the implant is made has to be biocompatible with the host tissues (bone and soft tissue) into which the implant is being placed to ensure that osseointegration occurs. Implants have been made of various materials. In the early 1990s implants made from aluminium oxide (ceramic) (see Fig. 2.4) were used to replace single teeth. Because of the brittle nature of the material, the implants failed as a result of fracture of the material and caused significant problems with infection and subsequent removal.

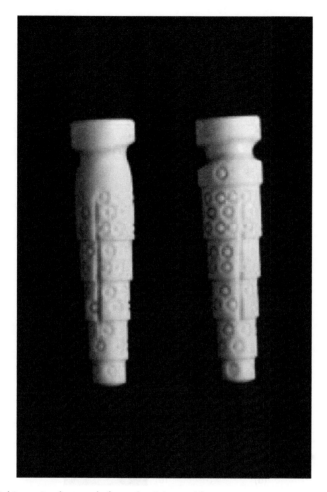

Figure 2.4   Tubingen implant made from aluminium oxide

Commercially pure titanium has been shown to have excellent biocom-patibility with the oral environment. The second-generation osseointegrated dental implants are made of commercially pure titanium and when exposed to air a thin oxide layer forms on the outer surface of the implant. This layer is crucial in determining the biological response of the host once the implant is placed into the bone. Although the majority of the implant systems available on the market today are made of commercially pure titanium, some of the systems with newer configurations contain small amounts of alloy within the internal connection of the implant to facilitate durability for the prosthetic connection. This alloy content to date has not been shown to have any adverse effects on the success rate of the implant.

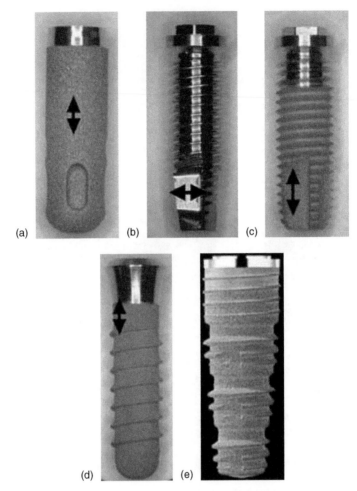

Figure 2.5 (a) Cylindrical parallel-sided fixture (IMZ). (b), (c), (d) Screw implants (also called threaded implants), which are parallel sided: (b) Brånemark implant, (c) osseotite (3i) implant, (d) Straumann implant. (e) Tapered screw design implant (Frialit 2)

Design

The design of the implant is crucial in determining its stability once it has been placed in bone. The main designs used today are cylindrical or threaded (screw) implants (see Figs 2.5a–e).

Cylindrical implants do not have a screw thread on the outside of the implant and are inserted into the prepared site as a 'press-fit' mechanism (see Fig. 2.5a). In contrast the threaded or screw-form implants are screwed into the jaw bone and therefore offer better primary stability (see Figs 2.5b–d). Today screw-form implants are the most universally used. Tapered or root-form implants shaped to resemble the root of the tooth are also available in either of the above configurations and are designed mainly for use immediately after tooth extraction because they are shaped like the root of the tooth (see Fig. 2.5e). These tapered implants are more technique sensitive and have also been used where the bone width has been compromised due to a narrow apical diameter. The majority of implant systems market the screw design (either tapered or standard) and the cylindrical designs are less popular. Some of the newer designs of implants have incorporated a combination of the tapered design coronally (to facilitate close proximity to the bone surface) and the screw-form design apically. These implants have been designed to replace teeth immediately following extraction so that the wider coronal aspect of the implant can be engaged into the coronal jaw bone, for example the Straumann tapered effect (TE) fixture.

Surface condition of the implant

The surface condition of the implant is very important for the bone to implant contact. The first implants to emerge were made of pure machined surfaces (see Fig. 2.6).

With these surfaces, the healing period required for osseointegration ranged from 4 months in the mandible to 6 months in the maxilla, where the bone is slightly less dense. To improve the osseointegration, surface-coated implants, in which the outer surface of the machined implant was coated with a bioactive material such as hydroxyapatite, were made available (Calciteck implants). Although in the early stages these implants showed good integration, with time it was shown that disintegration of the surface coating led to healing by fibrous

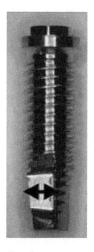

Figure 2.6 Fixture with a pure machined surface

tissue and subsequent failure of the implants. It is now known that if the topography of the implant surface is altered to increase the area into which the bone cells can penetrate, osseointegration can occur much faster. This concept was utilized in the third generation of implants in which the implant surface was either plasma sprayed or acid etched (see Figs 2.7a–c).This change in surface topography has enabled healing periods for osseointegration to be reduced to as little as 8 weeks. More recently advances in nanotechnology have resulted in newer surface topographies, called the nanotopography, which enable osseointegration to occur within 4 weeks, giving rise to the fourth-generation titanium implants. The majority of systems today provide surfaces with topographies aimed at increasing the surface area, thereby shortening the time period over which osseointegration of the implant to the jaw bone occurs. The current focus is on reducing healing times for osseointegration.

Factors relating to the host

Status of the host bed

The health of the host bed (the bone and the soft tissues) into which the implant is placed is important in determining how quickly and how well the implant will osseointegrate. The amount of blood in the bone site (called the vascularity) and the quality of the bone into which the implant is being placed are crucial factors that determine how well the implant will integrate into the jaw bone. The vascularity determines how many bone cells are available to help with the osseointegration process. If the blood supply is reduced or compromised, then the rate at which osseointegration can occur will be affected due to the reduced number of cells that can be transformed into bone-forming cells. The bone quality is assessed by the density of the bone, which is a ratio of the amount of cancellous bone to compact bone. The density of the bone is graded as type I to type IV, with type I bone being the most dense and type IV being the softest (see Fig. 2.8).

Dense bone is very hard and has fewer blood vessels. As this type of bone is hard, during preparation of the site for implant placement special additional drills, called screw taps, may need to be used to stop the bone from being overheated. The bone density also helps to determine the extent of initial stability (primary stability) and degree of movement in the initial healing period. The quality of the bone varies between the mandible and the maxilla, with the maxilla having softer bone than the mandible.

Surgical technique at the time of insertion

The predictability of osseointegration is dependant on ensuring that the site is not overheated during preparation (<47°C). The site is prepared sequentially

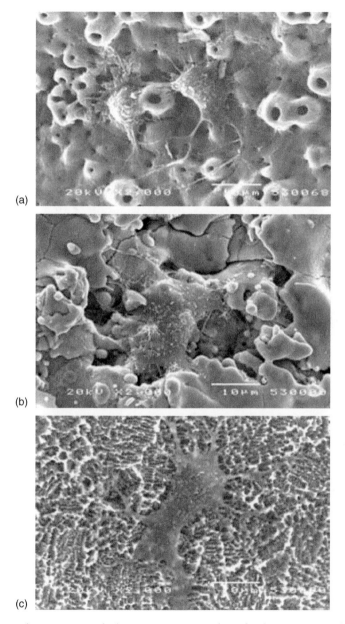

Figure 2.7   **(a)** Electronmicrograph showing a Ti-Unite surface. **(b)** Electronmicrograph showing a titanium plasma-sprayed surface. **(c)** Electronmicrograph showing acid-etched surface topography

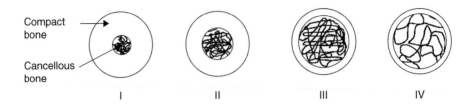

Figure 2.8   The different densities of bone, which are categorized as I (most dense, left) to IV (softest, right). The classification is based on the ratio of the cortical to the cancellous bone

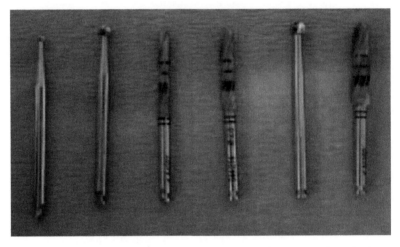

Figure 2.9   Range of drills used for the sequential preparation of the site to place the fixture

using sharp drills at slow speed and minimal pressure, starting from small round burs and going up to twist drills, which are used to prepare the site to the required width and depth. The drills increase in size gradually, with the final drill diameter being slightly smaller than the implant diameter (see Fig. 2.9). The site is prepared intermittently with copious water cooling to minimize the effects of the frictional heat generated during the drilling sequence. If the bone is overheated during the drilling sequence, then bone necrosis will occur, leading to failure of the implant.

Loading conditions applied afterwards

Loading of the implants can be undertaken at either four or six months after the implant placement (delayed loading), 1–2 months after placement (early loading) or immediately after placing the implants on the same day. The first option is chosen when the there is a compromise in the host site during placement and any risk of loading early would cause failure. Early loading has become possible with third-generation implants due to the changes in the surface topography of the implants screws, and should be undertaken only when there is good primary stability of the implant in the bone in which it is placed. Immediate loading is still a relatively new concept and should only be undertaken when all factors, such as primary stability, implant length and occlusion, are favourable. In compromised sites, premature loading of the implants can lead to early failure as a result of fibrous tissue formation.

Dental implant components

A restoration retained with a dental implant is made of two main components (see Fig. 2.10):

- the **screw** (also called the fixture or implant), which has to be placed surgically into the bone with the intent of achieving osseointegration. The implants can have different surfaces, as discussed earlier, to enhance osseointegration.
- the **prosthetic component**, which comprises of the abutments and screws. The abutment connects directly to the top of the implant and extends through the gingivae to the oral cavity. A screw, called the **abutment screw,** is used to connect the abutment to the implant. The crown is then either screwed onto the abutment with a prosthetic screw or cemented onto the abutment. Sometimes the crown and abutment can be made in one piece and screwed directly into the implant. The fitting surface of the abutments will contain a matching hex surface that enables accurate seating of the

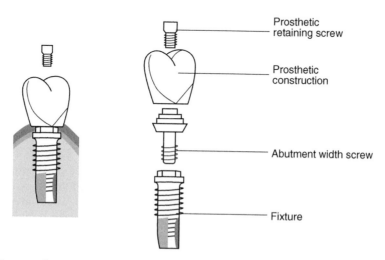

Figure 2.10   Different component parts of the implant retained restoration

abutment onto the implant. Implants with different types of connections will have abutments which match the type of connection. The abutments are also available in different sizes and configurations.

The fixture (screw)

The design of the fixture can vary and may be parallel sided, tapered or a combination and has been discussed previously. Irrespective of the design the concepts and function of the screw remain the same. The screw will also have features in the apical part to facilitate insertion into the bone. The top of the screw onto which the prosthesis fits is called the 'platform'. The implants come in different diameters to match different sizes of teeth (3.25–6.00 mm). This enables the crown to be made to match the tooth being replaced so that the best emergence profile for the prosthesis can be achieved. The exact diameters vary between the different systems but nearly all will have a narrow diameter to cater for small teeth, such as upper lateral incisors and lower central incisors, a regular platform to cater for normal-sized teeth, such as upper central incisors, premolars and canines, and a wide platform to cater for the larger sized teeth, such as the molars and occasionally the canine teeth (see Figs 2.11a–c).

The implant screws also come in different lengths, with the shortest being 6 mm and the longest being up to 15 mm. In the past screw lengths of up to 20 mm were also available; however, today it is rare to use lengths longer than 15 mm because of the changes in surface topography that allow better and more predictable integration (see Fig. 2.12).

The screw platform can have two types of connection within the coronal aspect by which the prosthesis is connected into the screw. The role of the connection is also to prevent rotation of the prosthetic components when they are fitted. This connection can be:

- an **external connection** in which the connection extends out on top of the platform, and can be an octagon or a hexagon. The latter is often referred to as an 'external hex' (see Fig. 2.13) or
- an **internal connection** in which the connection sits within the coronal third of the screw. This type of connection is available in different designs can be hexagonal or a morse taper. In the latter the internal connection interface consists of a converging circular surface that forms a mechanical interlock (see Figs 2.14a, b)

The screw part of the implant is placed surgically into the bone under sterile conditions. Depending on the clinical indications the fixture platform is then protected with either a cover screw or a healing abutment, both of which aim to stop the bone and soft tissue from growing into the fixture. The healing abutment is normally used when the fixture is to be left exposed in the mouth, called the one-stage procedure. The cover screw is used when the fixture is to be embedded under the gingival tissue for a period of time, called a two-stage procedure. A second surgical procedure is then necessary to remove the cover screw and

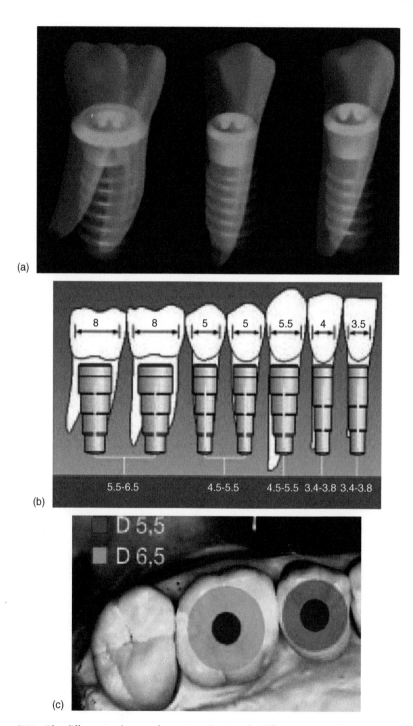

Figure 2.11   The different implant configurations showing the different implant diameters in relation to the size of the teeth

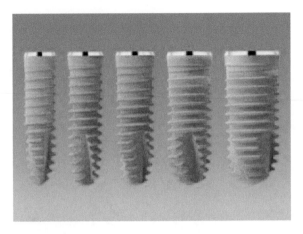

Figure 2.12   Different lengths of XiVe fixtures, ranging from 7 to 18 mm

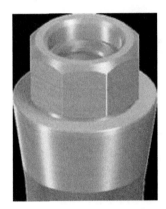

Figure 2.13   The external hex connection where the hexagon projects above the top surface of the fixture

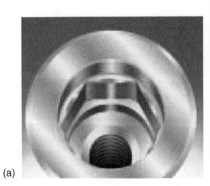

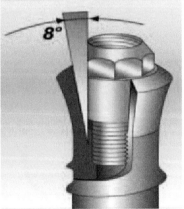

(a)   (b)

Figure 2.14   **(a)** The internal connection fixture with the configurate which helps impart accurate seating. This configuration varies with different systems. **(b)** The 8° morse taper for interlocking

replace it with a healing abutment. The healing abutment comes in different shapes and helps to remodel the gingival tissue in preparation for taking the impressions for the prosthetic construction. The details of the surgical procedure are covered in Chapter 3. The majority of systems have a separate surgical kit that is used to place the fixture in the jaw bone.

The prosthetic components

The prosthetic components are made up of two aspects: the components that are used clinically and those that are required by the laboratory to construct the implant-retained crown, bridge or denture. This chapter only covers the laboratory components that are clinically relevant for the nurse.

Clinical components

Abutment
The abutment, as discussed earlier, retains the prosthesis on the fixture and connects directly into it. The abutment can be custom made (see Fig. 2.15a), prefabricated (machined) (see Fig. 2.15b) or temporary (see Fig. 2.15c).

A temporary abutment is used to fabricate a temporary prosthesis. Machined abutments are made of titanium, gold or ceramic and are simple to use, requiring minimal chair-side time. The choice of the abutment is dependent on the type

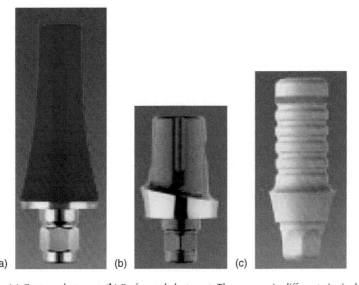

(a)   (b)   (c)

Figure 2.15   **(a)** Custom abutment. **(b)** Preformed abutment. These come in different gingival heights. **(c)** Temporary abutment. The abutments shown are those for the Friadent XiVe implant system

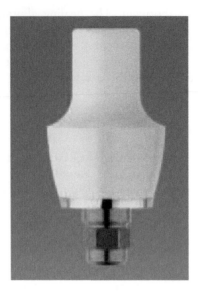

Figure 2.16   Ceramic abutment, which is cut to the required shape to construct the crown

of prosthesis being made, for example crown, bridge or denture. Abutments can be connected directly into the mouth in the laboratory. If the abutment is connected in the mouth, a protective cap, called a healing cap, needs to be placed onto the abutment to protect it in the mouth whilst the prosthesis is being constructed. A custom abutment can be prepared to the required shape in the laboratory or can be made by computer-aided design–computer-aided manufacture (CAD-CAM). This abutment is supplied as a blank in either titanium or ceramic for the clinician or technician to prepare to the required dimensions (see Fig. 2.16).

Different types of screws are required to connect the abutment and the prosthesis to the implant. The screws available are:

- **abutment fixture screws:** used to screw the abutment into the fixture. Once used the screw will need to be tightened ('torqued') to the correct level to ensure that the abutment does not come loose from the implant. The torque can be applied using a machine or, more commonly, a hand-held torque driver.
- **prosthetic screws:** used to retain the prosthesis, for example the crown or bridge, in the abutment if the restoration is going to be screw retained. These are also called retaining screws.

Impression coping

This is a device used to register and transfer the clinical information about the position of the implant fixture or the abutment and the soft tissues in the mouth to the laboratory technician. There are two different types of impression copings: the fixture level coping (or the pick up impression coping) and the transfer

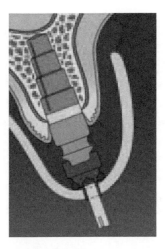

Figure 2.17 Open impression technique where the screw of the impression coping projects out of the tray

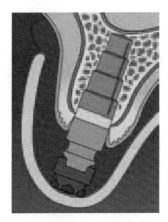

Figure 2.18 Closed impression technique where the impression coping is enclosed in the impression tray

impression coping. With the former an open impression tray is used. This allows access to the retaining screw that connects the impression coping to the fixture (see Fig. 2.17). Once the impression material is set, the screw is loosened and the whole impression, with the impression coping and the retaining screw, is taken out of the mouth. The laboratory analogue is then attached to the coping before the model is poured up. For the transfer coping, the impression coping is connected to the implant in the mouth and an impression taken using a closed technique (see Fig. 2.18). Once set the impression is removed and the coping remains on the implant. This then needs to be unscrewed and seated back into

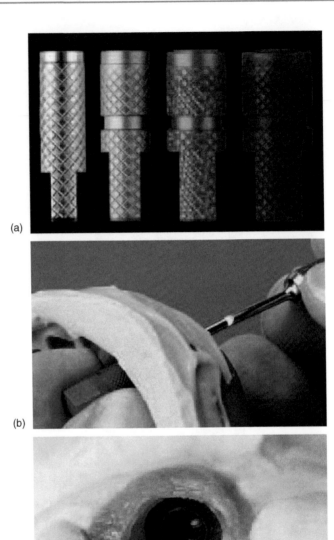

Figure 2.19 **(a)** Fixture analogues of different sizes. The analogues are colour coded to match the different implant diameters. **(b)** The fixture analogue being connected into the impression. **(c)** Model showing the fixture analogue in situ

the impression. The technician will then connect the fixture analogue to the coping. Transfer copings should only be used when the fixtures are placed in perfect alignment and there is no divergence. If the fixtures point in different directions then open tray impression should be used. Abutment level impression copings are used as either closed or open techniques. The abutment has to be selected first and connected in the mouth and torqued prior to the impression being taken. The impression coping is then placed onto the abutment and an impression taken. On removal of the impression, the abutment is left connected to the implant in the mouth and a healing cap is placed on it to protect it. The abutment level impression coping comes away in the impression. The technician connects the abutment replica to the coping before pouring the model. This is then used to construct the definitive restoration.

Laboratory components

Fixture (implant) analogue
This is a copy of the implant fixture that is placed into the jaw bone. Fixture analogues come in the same sizes as implant fixtures (see Fig. 2.19a). The technician places the fixture analogue into the impression and makes a master model of the impression. This model is then used to construct the implant-retained prosthesis (see Figs 2.19a–c).

Abutment replica
This is a copy of the abutment which is used to construct the prosthesis.

Retaining/prosthetic screws
These are screws that are used during the construction of the prosthesis to retain it on the cast.

Gold cylinders
These are laboratory components that are machined to fit onto the abutments. Implant restorations should be made with metal that is compatible with the implant components. Noble metal alloys are usually used in implant restorations because base metal alloys have a much higher melting point.

Implant systems 3

Implantology to date has enjoyed a progressive, albeit rapid, development, with over 250 implant systems with different designs and features available on the market. Some of these systems are well researched with documented evidence of their success; others, however, have little or no published data to support them. This rapid expansion has been driven by patient as well as clinician demand as the predictability and success rates of endoosseous dental implants have improved. In response to these demands, different companies have competed to introduce products aimed at achieving shorter treatment times and improved aesthetics, thus enabling teeth to be replaced in a day. Chapter 2 provided an overview of the concepts of osseointegration and the components of modern-day implantology. This chapter focuses on five of the more commonly used implant systems. Although there are minor variations in the names of products and components used by different companies, the basic concepts remain the same. An overview of the basic outline of the systems is given; however, the different types of motors used for surgical procedures are not covered.

The systems

The systems covered are:

- the Brånemark System® marketed by Nobelbiocare
- the Straumann System marketed by Straumann
- the Frialit 2, XiVe and Ankylos systems marketed by Dentsply Friadent

- the 3i System marketed by Implant Innovations
- the Astra System marketed by Astra Tech.

We will focus on the different components of the systems and the key differences between them. Each system has three main categories of product line: the surgical components, prosthetic components and the instrumentation needed for the implant placement and restoration. All the systems also have different types of planning kits, the details of which are beyond the scope of this chapter.

The Brånemark System®

This was the first osseointegrated implant system that was to receive worldwide recognition and it has today changed the way endoosseous implant treatment is undertaken. This system was first introduced in 1980 with a kit that enabled the placement of dental implants into the jaw bone of edentulous patients to support dentures. The fixtures that were supplied at the time were designed by Professor Brånemark in conjunction with one of his co-workers and were first marketed under the name of Nobelpharma in 1982. This company established stringent manufacturing criteria and produced the first products in 1982, which were used by practitioners. In 1985 the company changed its name to Nobel Industries and the Brånemark System® was named as such in 1990. Subsequently, when the company took over the Sterioss implant system, the name changed to Nobelbiocare. Today the two implant systems marketed by this company are the Brånemark System® and the Replace Select System. The latter is the internal connection system that is marketed by the company and at present appears to be taking over the market share of the Brånemark System®. This chapter will only cover the Brånemark System®.

When it was first marketed, the Brånemark System® followed stringent protocols of design and equipment. Whilst the early equipment was cumbersome and complex, the system has now been streamlined, with a significant reduction in the number of instruments and drivers needed both for the surgical and the prosthetic aspects of treatment. Over the past 20 years, the system has seen a vast change in the product line, with different types of implants available for different situations.

Implants

The company provides fixtures for extra-oral as well as intra-oral use. This chapter focuses on the intra-oral components. The implants for intra-oral use have an external hex connection and are designed as parallel-walled implants with an apical cutting flute that minimizes trauma during placement (see Fig. 3.1).

The implants are provided in a range of lengths from 7 to 20 mm; however, the most commonly used lengths today range from 10 to 15 mm. The implants are available in a choice of diameters, with the smallest being 3.3 mm – the

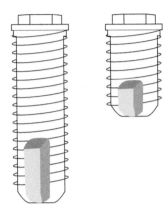

Figure 3.1 Brånemark fixtures with the apical self-cutting thread and the external hex connection

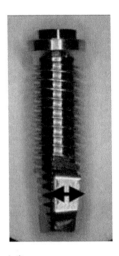

Figure 3.2 Pure machined Brånemark fixture

narrow platform (NP); the 3.75 and 4 mm diameters – the regular platform (RP) and finally 5.0 and 6.0 mm diameters, the wide platform (WP). Recently the company has introduced a short 5.5 mm length implant called the 'shorty', which is also available in all the diameters.

All the fixtures are available as Mark III implants for use in all types of bone and as Mark IV fixtures primarily designed for use in type IV bone. The surface finish of the implants was originally a pure machined titanium surface (see Fig. 3.2), but today this surface has been superseded by the Ti-Unite® surface. The implant surface topography is changed by putting the implant through an oxidation process, which results in a porous and thicker titanium oxide layer. It is this layer that increases the surface area over which the bone cells can grow and integrate (see Fig. 3.3).

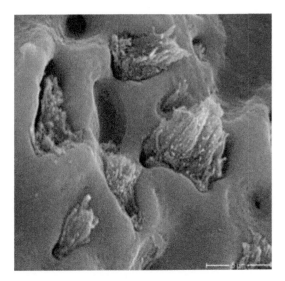

Figure 3.3 Electronmicrograph showing the Ti-Unite surface, which is prepared by an oxidation process that results in a porous and thicker titanium oxide layer

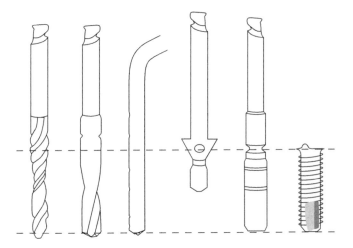

Figure 3.4 The drilling protocol of the Brånemark system

The original implants marketed as Mark II had to be tapped into place using a screw tap. This soon changed with the introduction of the Mark III implants, which were self-tapping with the special cutting thread apically. The drilling sequence for the site preparation remains similar to that discussed in Chapter 2 (see Fig. 3.4). A pilot drill was used in the original drilling protocol, but this seems to have been eliminated from the recent drilling protocol. The company produced disposable one-use-only drills to eliminate the repeated use of

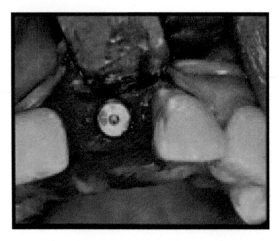

Figure 3.5   Clinical picture of a Brånemark fixture in situ showing the external hex at the level of the alveolar crest

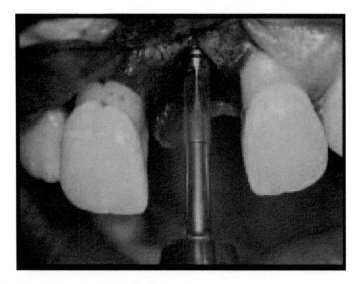

Figure 3.6   Fixture being placed with the fixture driver

blunt drills, which could overheat the bone and compromise the site preparation and ultimate success of the fixtures. The final step in the site preparation is the use of the countersink or 'counterbore' as it is now called. This is used to enable the implant to be placed such that the external hex connection sits in line with the alveolar crest (see Fig. 3.5). The first implants were premounted, and once placed the fixture mounts had to be removed. This step has now been eliminated with the implant driver being designed such that the implant can be picked up directly, eliminating the need to remove the fixture mount (see Fig. 3.6).

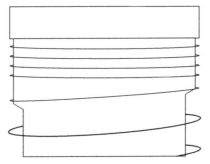

Figure 3.7   The groove fixture showing the threads extending higher up on the fixture

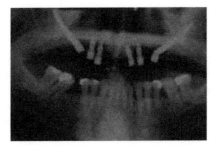

Figure 3.8   Zygoma implant

Position indicators and depth gauges are used to check the drilling depth and fixture alignment during site preparation. All the implants are supplied with a cover screw. The latest change within this system is the change in the configuration of the grooves on the implant surface. The threads are much higher up on the implant surface and extend onto the implant collar (see Fig. 3.7). The grooves have been incorporated to enable more rapid bone formation, thus enabling the implants to integrate faster. The grooves also provide a better mechanical interlock, improving primary stability. The system also has the 'zygoma' implant, which has similar features to the implants covered above (see Fig. 3.8).

The company has also introduced a number of other implants to the market to meet demand. Other implants that are being marketed are the 'nobelspeedy', which allows for flapless surgery and has a slight taper. Other concepts are 'implants in a day' (when the implants are inserted and the prosthesis is also connected at the same time so that patients leave the surgery with their teeth) and the 'nobelguide' treatment concept (where specially made customised surgical guide is used to transfer the planned treatment to the patients mouth such that an exact replica of the prosthesis is delivered).

Prosthetic components

The original Brånemark System® had a number of prosthetic components (see Fig. 3.9a). The first abutments were the standard abutment (see Fig. 3.9b), the ceraone abutment (see Fig. 3.9c), the aestheticone abutment (see Fig. 3.9d) and the mirus cone abutment for sites with minimal space. In addition two angulated abutments are also available. These are the preformed abutment and the custom abutment, a UCLA type (see Fig. 3.9e) is also available. The preformed abutments have now been replaced with multiunit abutments, which the company says are compatible with previous abutments (see Fig. 3.10). The system has impression copings for fixture level impressions as well as abutment level impressions (see Figs 3.11a, b). The abutments screws are tightened to a torque of 20 Ncm and the prosthetic screws to a torque of 10 Ncm, with the exception of the ceraone abutment screw, which should be tightened to 35 Ncm.

Instrumentation

The cumbersome equipment that was needed for implant surgery when first introduced was replaced in the mid-1990s with compact and more user-friendly instrumentation kits (see Figs 3.12a, b). The kits of today are colour coded and extensively simplified, thus making them easier to use. The kits available are the surgical kit, the second-stage surgery kit and the prosthetic kit. The torque drivers were originally machine driven, but the hand-held torque driver has now largely replaced the old machine-driven driver.

The Straumann System

This system is Swiss, with Straumann having an interest in metallurgy and precision mechanics. The company has close links with the International Team of Implantologists (ITI), a group that undertakes independent research in the field of implantology. The first implant, called the Boneloc implant, was developed in the mid-1970s by Andre Shroeder and his team. This was a hollow cylinder implant and they confirmed that direct bone to implant contact can occur under the correct conditions. As a result of this finding, in 1985 the one-part and two-part hollow cylinder and hollow screw fixtures (implants) were manufactured. Because of problems with fracture, the hollow cylinder implants were subsequently replaced in the early 1990s by the solid screw implants.

Implants

The company provides implants for extra-oral and intra-oral use and they also have an orthodontic implant. The fixture is designed as a cylindrical implant with an internal octagon connection, which also has a morse taper. The morse taper provides the antirotation with a reliable and stable implant-to-abutment joint, whereas the internal octagon confers flexibility but also ensures accurate

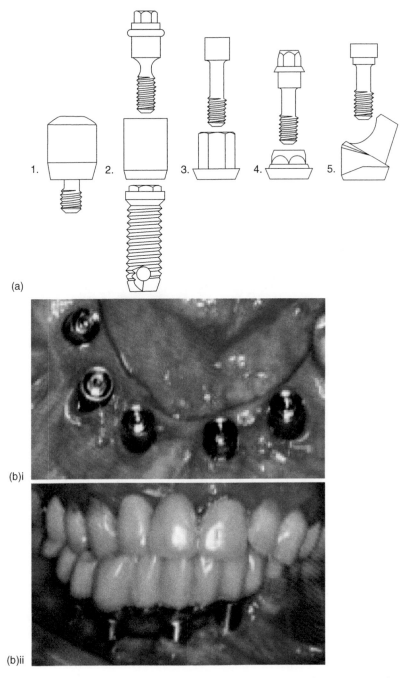

(a)

(b)i

(b)ii

Figure 3.9 **(a)** 1, healing abutment; 2, standard abutment; 3, ceraone abutment; 4, aestheticone abutment; 5, angulated abutment. **(b)** **(i, ii)** Standard abutments in clinical use retaining a fixed prosthesis.

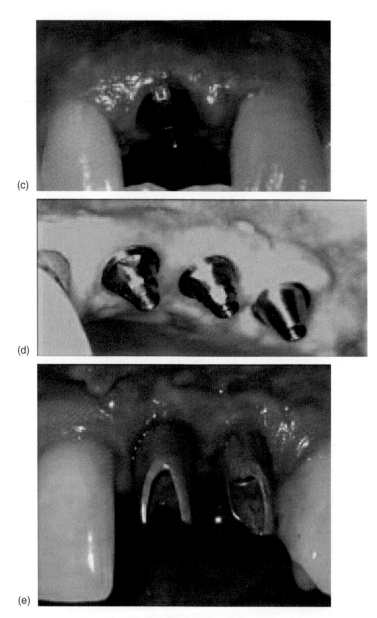

(c)

(d)

(e)

Figure 3.9 *Continued*   **(c)** Ceraone abutment used for the replacement of a single tooth. **(d)** The aestheticone abutments used for replacing multiple teeth. **(e)** Custom abutment seated in the mouth

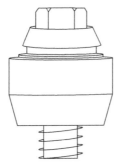

Figure 3.10 The multiunit abutment

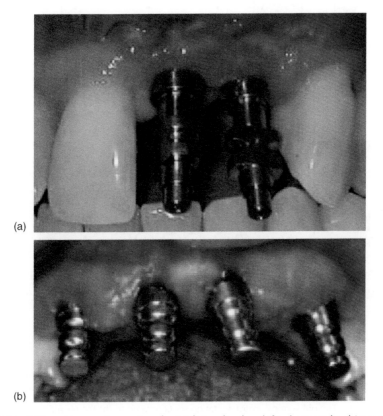

(a)

(b)

Figure 3.11 Different impression copings for **(a)** fixture level and **(b)** abutment level impressions

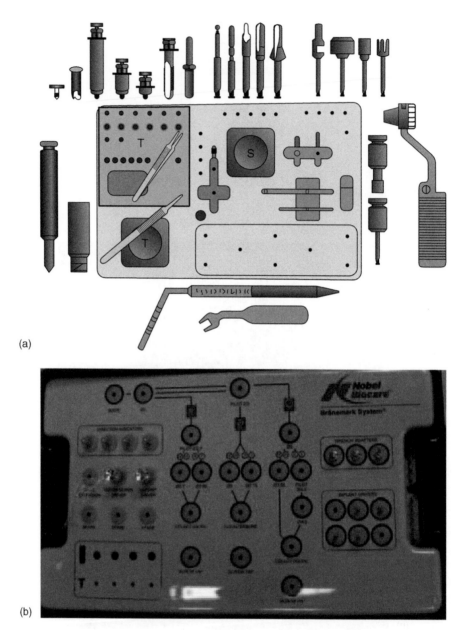

(a)

(b)

Figure 3.12 (a) The old surgical instrumentation set compared to (b) the newer set

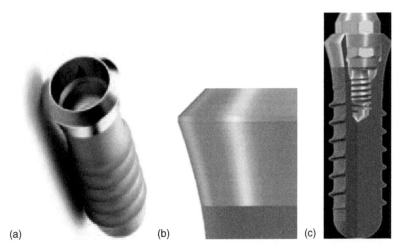

(a) (b) (c)

Figure 3.13 **(a)** Straumann fixture showing the internal connection. **(b)** The bevel that minimizes the microgap and allows for optimal load distribution. **(c)** The 8° Morse taper that provides the anti-rotation and a stable implant to abutment join

repositioning of the prosthesis. The 45° beveled shoulder allows for optimal load distribution and minimizes the microgap between the implant and the prosthesis. Primarily designed for use as a one-stage system, the main difference with this system is that the implants have the polished collar integrated into the body of the implant, which allows for soft tissue adaptation during healing after the surgical placement of the implant (see Figs 3.13a, b, c).

The implants are provided in a range of lengths, starting at 6 mm with the longest being 16 mm. The most commonly used are the 10–12 mm lengths. The 6 mm implant is only used when it is connected to other implants. The family of implants is available in three lines: standard, standard plus and tapered effect (TE) (Fig. 3.14). The main difference between the standard and standard plus implants is the height of the polished collar. The standard implant has a 2.8 mm polished collar whereas with the standard plus (previously called the aesthetic plus) the polished collar is reduced to 1.8 mm. This implant is advocated for use mainly in the aesthetic areas. The TE fixture has a special design and is advocated for used for immediate implantation. It has a slight coronal flare, which is thought to confer better primary stability by engaging the cortical plate coronally. All the implants are available in a choice of three diameters: the narrow body of 3.3 mm diameter, the regular body with a 4.1 mm diameter and the wide body with a 4.8 mm diameter (see Figs 3.15a, b, c).

The prosthetic platform diameters are, however, different and are available as 3.5 mm diameter (narrow neck, NN), 4.8 mm diameter (regular neck, RN) and 6.5 mm (wide neck, WN) diameter (see Figs 3.16a, b, c). The narrow neck, because of its size, is an external connection and is only available on the narrow body implant (3.3 mm). The regular neck is available on the narrow body

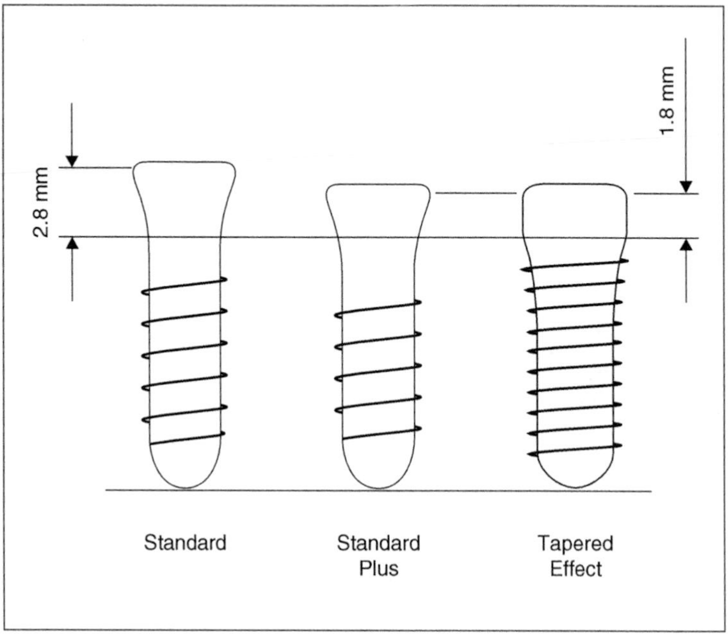

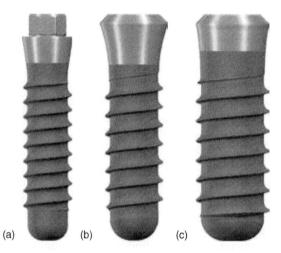

Figure 3.14   The family of Straumann fixtures showing the standard, standard plus and tapered effect fixtures

Figure 3.15   **(a)** The narrow body fixture with a 3.3 mm diameter, **(b)** a regular body fixture with a 4.1 mm diameter and **(c)** a wide body diameter of 4.8 mm

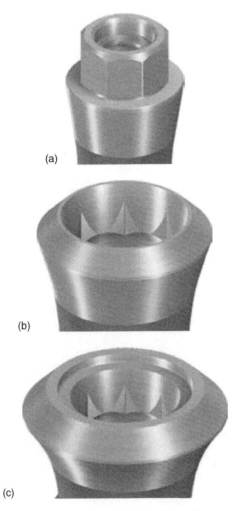

(a)

(b)

(c)

Figure 3.16 The different range of prosthetic diameters from **(a)** 3.5 mm as the narrow neck, **(b)** 4.8 mm as the regular neck and **(c)** 6.5 mm as the wide neck. Note that the narrow neck fixture has an external octogon connection

(3.3 mm), regular body (4.1 mm) and wide body (4.8 mm). The wide neck is only available on the wide body (4.8 mm).

The original implant surface was titanium plasma sprayed (TPS) (see Fig. 3.17) and needed up to 12 weeks for integration to occur. To meet the market needs of shorter healing times this surface was replaced with the sand-blasted large grit acid-etched (SLA) surface in 1994 (see Fig. 3.18). The implant was put through a process of large grit sand blasting with a conundrum of particles and then acid etched with hydrochloric and sulphuric acid to create micropits on the implant surface. These micropits were associated with improved integration and

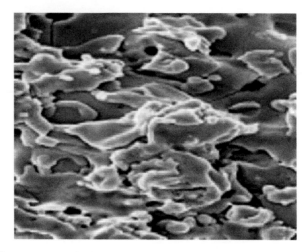

Figure 3.17 Electronmicrograph showing the titanium plasma-sprayed surface of the Straumann implant

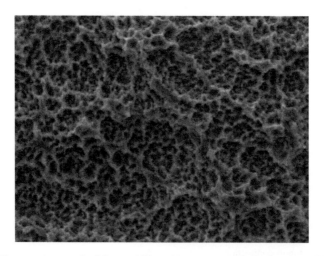

Figure 3.18 Electronmicrograph of the sand-blasted large grit acid-etched surface of the Straumann implant. Note the difference compared to the previous implant in the surface area. The SLA active surface is an enhanced surface of the SLA aimed at improving the osseointegration rate

shorter healing times, reducing the healing time for the implant to integrate to 6–8 weeks. More recently this surface has been modified again and implants with an SLA active surface have been introduced. This is a hydroxilated (chemically active) surface, which provides ideal conditions for direct protein absorption and thus immediate initiation of osseointegration. This macro- and microstructured osseoconductive surface therefore reduces the healing times for integration to 3–4 weeks.

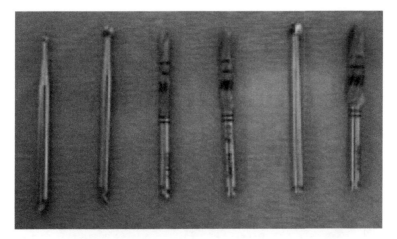

Figure 3.19 The Straumann round and twist drills used for site preparation. Note the black markings on the twist drills, which indicate the depth to which the site is being prepared

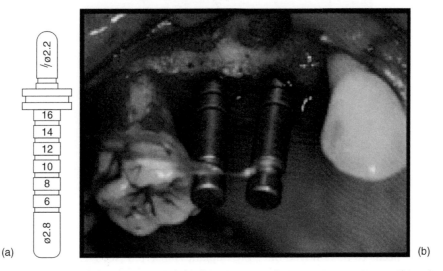

(a) (b)

Figure 3.20 **(a)** The alignment pin and **(b)** the pins in situ during site preparation, verifying the fixture position

The drilling sequence of the implants remains the same as detailed in Chapter 2, but for the standard plus implants a profile drill (similar to the countersink) needs to be used for the emergence profile. With the TE implant a cortical drill has to be used to facilitate the preparation of the coronal part of the site to enable the tapered part of the implant to engage the cortical bone. Fig. 3.19 shows the drill sequence (the profile drill is not included in this figure). This system has depth gauges, which are also used as direction indicators and are called 'alignment pins' (see Figs 3.20a, b). The fixtures are pre-mounted and the

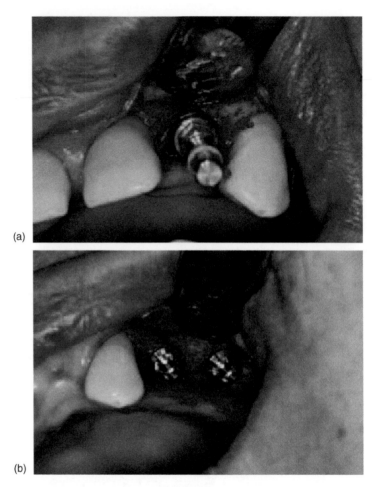

(a)

(b)

Figure 3.21   The fixture mounts **(a)** in situ and **(b)** after removal

mount needs to be removed once the implant is inserted (see Figs 3.21a, b). The other implants available are the extra-oral (see Fig. 3.22) and the orthodontic implants, which can be used for anchorage when there is an inadequate number of teeth (see Fig. 3.23).

Prosthetic components

This system has three categories of abutments: the solid abutment (see Fig. 3.24a), the synocta abutment (see Fig. 3.24b) and the angulated abutment (see Fig. 3.24c). The abutments for narrow neck implants are different and have an external connection. The abutments are available both for cementable and screw-retained restorations. The same screw driver (see Fig. 3.25) is used for all prosthetic parts. The abutments are screwed into the implant and torqued to

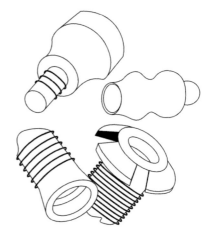

Figure 3.22 Extra-oral Straumann implant

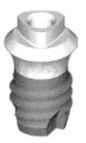

Figure 3.23 Orthodontic Straumann implant, which is used in cases where there is an inadequate number of teeth for anchorage

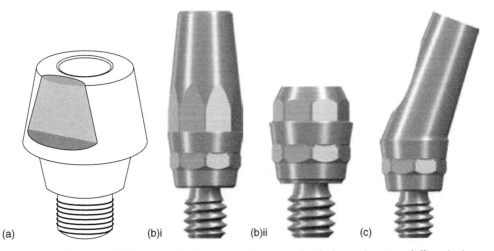

(a)   (b)i   (b)ii   (c)

Figure 3.24 **(a)** Solid abutment. **(b)** The synocta abutments for **(i)** the single unit and **(ii)** multiple unit restorations. The former is designed with antirotation to stop the abutment from rotating on the fixture. **(c)** Angled abutment

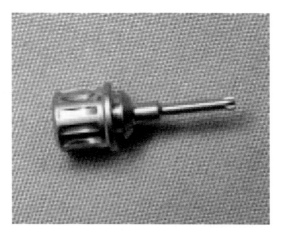

Figure 3.25   Standard screw driver, which is used for all prosthetic connections with the exception of the locator and ball and socket abutments

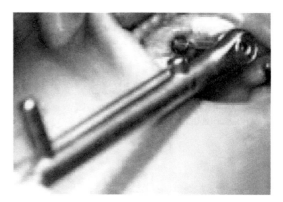

Figure 3.26   Manual torque wrench used to tighten the abutment and prosthetic screws

35 Ncm using a manual torque driver (see Fig. 3.26). The prosthetic screws for the screw-retained restoration are torqued to 15 Ncm. The impression copings are called transfer caps and are available for use at fixture or abutment level. The caps are available in metal or with a white plastic basket and positioning cylinder for both the implant (see Figs 3.27a, b) and abutment level impressions (see Figs 3.28a–e). Once the impression has been taken the analogues are positioned and the cast is poured for the construction of the prosthesis.

Instrumentation

The surgical tray is colour coded with the coloured lines showing the drilling sequence (see Fig. 3.29). The arrowed lines make it easy for nurses to find the

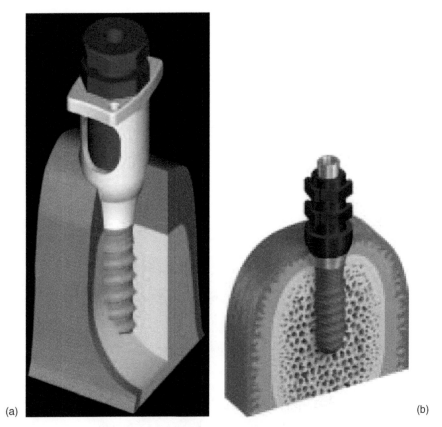

Figure 3.27 **(a)** White basket and red positioning cylinder fixture level transfer cap. **(b)** Metal screw fixture level impression coping

next component that is needed during site preparation. The prosthetic kit is also compact because only one screw driver and one torque driver are needed.

The Frialit 2 and XiVe systems

The Frialit 2 and XiVe are German systems and the implants were originally marketed by Friadent in the UK but have been bought over by Dentsply (in 2000). The Frialit®-1 implant, also known as the Tubigen implant, was made from aluminium oxide and initiated under the leadership of Professor Dr Willi Schulte in 1974. The concept behind this implant was to design it as a root-form implant, so that it could be immediately inserted into the bone at the time the tooth was extracted. The original ceramic implant was replaced in 1992 with the Frialit 2 (F2) implant because of problems with fracture and failure. Since the introduction of this implant, newer implant lines have been introduced.

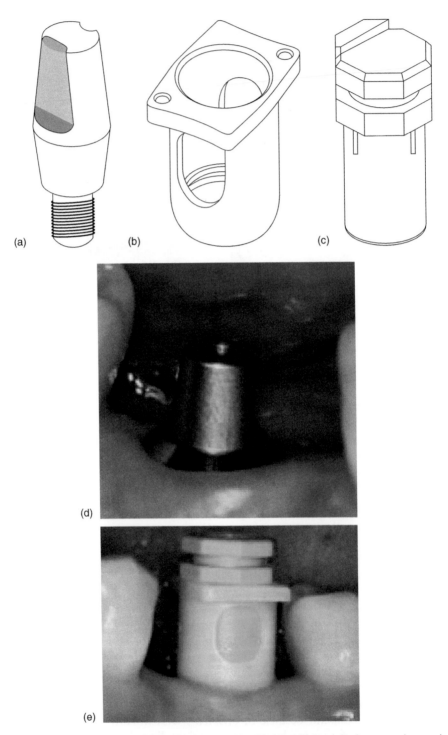

(a)   (b)   (c)   (d)   (e)

Figure 3.28 **(a–e)** Abutment level impression coping. The positioning cylinders are colour coded to match the solid abutment heights

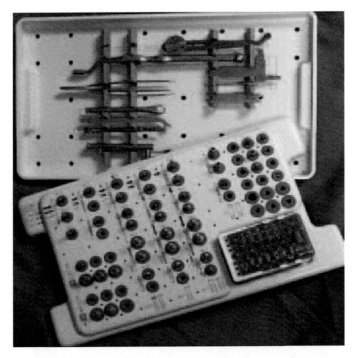

Figure 3.29 Surgical kit showing the coloured arrowed lines that indicate the drilling sequence

Although the IMZ implant is still around, its use has largely diminished and it will therefore not be covered here. This was the first implant system that used colour coding for easy identification of the different component parts.

Implants

F2 implants are available as root analogue stepped cylinders or stepped screws (see Fig. 3.30). The XiVe fixture (see Fig. 3.31) was introduced in 2003 as a parallel-sided implant with slight changes in the design to achieve the highest primary stability in all bone qualities. This was achieved by changing the apical thread configuration to deeper threads and incorporating a slightly wider crestal part to facilitate improved primary stability. The implants are made from commercially pure titanium and are designed with the same internal configuration connection as each other (see Fig. 3.32).

The fixtures have a precut thread to facilitate ease during placement, thus eliminating the need for a screw tap. The implants also have a polished collar coronally to provide flexibility for use as either a one or two-stage placement.

The F2 fixtures are available in four lengths (8, 11, 13 and 15 mm) and four diameters (3.5, 4.5, 5.5 and 6.5 mm) to match the diameter of the tooth that is

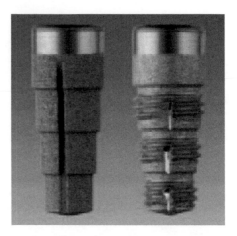

Figure 3.30   The Frialit 2® stepped push fit and screw implants

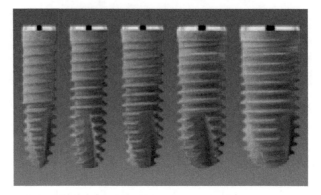

Figure 3.31   The XiVe® implant with the more pronounced threads apically and slightly wider crestal diameter to offer improved stability when placed

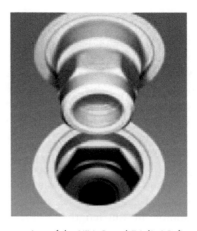

Figure 3.32   The internal connection of the XiVe® and Frialit 2® fixtures

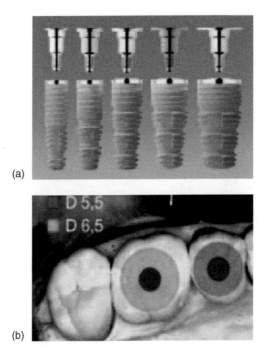

(a)

(b)

Figure 3.33 **(a)** The range of diameters with colour-coded cover screws. **(b)** The colour coding showing the relationship of the diameter to the size of the tooth

being replaced (see Figs 3.33a, b). The XiVe fixtures are available in lengths of 8–18 mm and diameters of 3.0–5.5 mm (see Fig. 3.34a). Each diameter configuration is colour coded with the colour scheme applied throughout the whole range of components (surgical to prosthetic) for that particular diameter (see Fig. 3.34b).

The original surface of the implant was a titanium plasma-sprayed surface (see Fig. 3.35), which was replaced by a deep profile, grit-blasted acid-etched surface. This surface has now been superseded by the 'cell plus' acid-etched surface (see Fig. 3.36), which shortens the healing time. Implant placement is undertaken using a series of standardized drills with internal irrigation. The drills for the F2 are stepped drills (see Fig. 3.37). The XiVe drilling sequence is the same, but an additional cortical drill has to be used to prepare the cortical part of the site (see Figs 3.38a, b, c).

Prosthetic components

The prosthetic components for the two systems are the same due to the same internal connection configuration. Different abutments are available and are either preformed (see Fig. 3.39) or customized. The latter is called the aurobase abutment (see Fig. 3.40). The prosthetic kit is compact, with a small range of screwdrivers needed for the prosthetic components (see Fig. 3.41). Once the

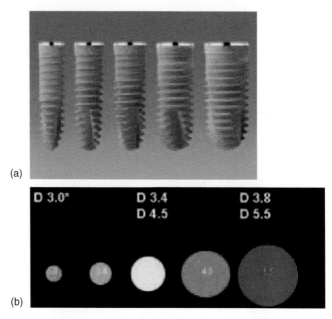

(a)

(b)

Figure 3.34 **(a)** The different diameters of the XiVe fixture. **(b)** The colour coding of the range of diameters

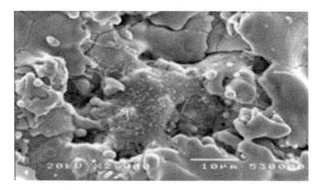

Figure 3.35 An electronmicrograph showing the titanium plasma-sprayed surface of the first range of fixtures

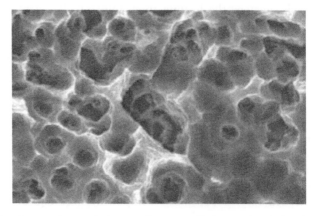

Figure 3.36 An electronmicrograph showing the new 'cell plus' acid-etched surface

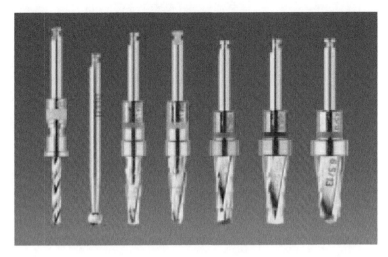

Figure 3.37   The stepped drills used for Frialit 2 site preparation. Note the colour-coded band

abutment is connected to the fixture, the abutment screws should be tightened to 20 Ncm and the prosthetic screws to 10 Ncm using a manual torque driver (see Fig. 3.42).

The impression copings are fixture level copings and have a plastic positioning sleeve that can be used to convert the coping for a closed tray (see Figs 3.43a, b). This sleeve also helps with the relocation of the coping into the impression. All the prosthetic components are also colour coded. The final prosthesis is fitted with a silicone ring, which provides a hermetic seal for the abutment and fixture. This seal is thought to prevent bacterial contamination (see Fig. 3.44).

Instrumentation

For both the F2 and the XiVe systems the surgical and the prosthetics kits are compact and each is colour coded (see Figs 3.45a, b). This system has a number of additional dummy implants, positioning cylinders and depth markers that can be used during the preparation for checking the alignment.

The Ankylos System

The Ankylos® implant system was developed by Professor Dr G-H Nentwig and Dr W Moser in 1985 and was made available for universal use in 1987. Their aim was to reproduce as closely as possible the prosthetic characteristics of the natural tooth. The implant was designed with a structure such that optimal load transmission was obtained during functional loading (see Fig. 3.46). The unique feature of this system is the conical connection of the prosthesis into the implant.

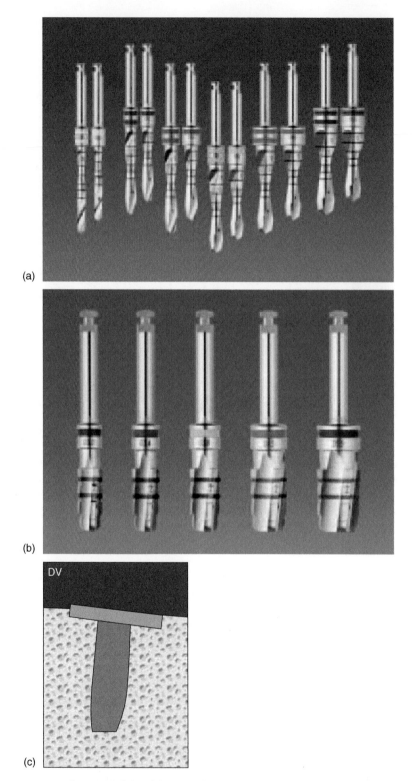

Figure 3.38 **(a)** The twist drills used for XiVe. **(b)** The special cortical drill used as the last drill to flare the cortical aspect of the site. **(c)** The flare after the use of the cortical drill in site preparation of the XiVe fixture

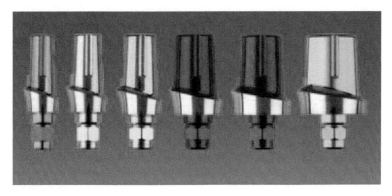

Figure 3.39 The preformed MH abutments

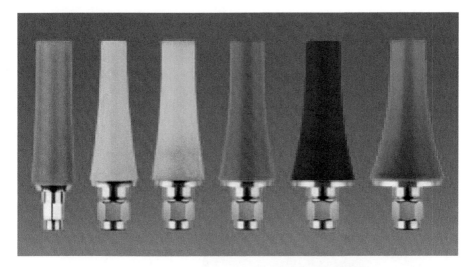

Figure 3.40 The custom aurobase abutments. Note the colour-coded sleeves

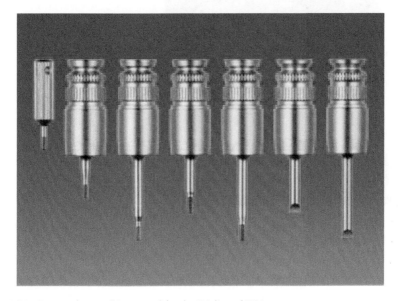

Figure 3.41 Range of screwdrivers used for the Frialit and XiVe systems

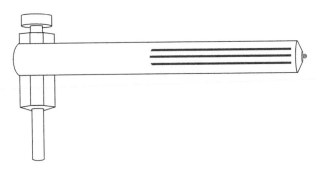

Figure 3.42 Manual torque driver

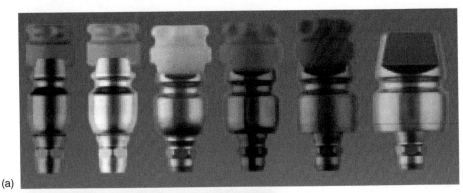

(a)

(b)

Figure 3.43 (**a**) Range of impression copings used at fixture level. Note the colour-coded plastic positioning sleeves. (**b**) Clinical picture showing the fixture level impression in situ with the colour-coded sleeve

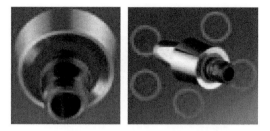

Figure 3.44 The blue silicone ring that is used to provide the hermetic seal at the fixture/abutment interface

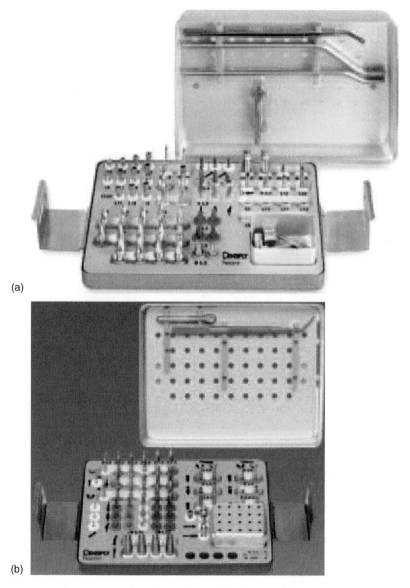

(a)

(b)

Figure 3.45 (a) The F2 surgical kit. The simplicity of the kit is evident. (b) The XiVe surgical kit

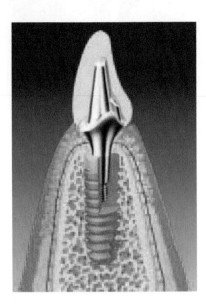

Figure 3.46   The unique design of the Ankylos system based on optimal load transmission during functional loading

This connection is thought to prevent microbial and mechanical irritation, thereby stabilizing the peri-implant hard and soft tissue. The system is primarily designed for intra-oral use.

Implants

Ankylos® implants are made from non-coated pure titanium. The implant thread is specially designed and progressively increases in depth apically, thus imparting greater stability in the bone (see Figs 3.47a, b). The implant has a unique internal connection with a precision surface fit of the conical connector at the implant/abutment interface (Fig. 3.48a, b). The very precise fit of the conical surface eliminates the microgap and hence the associated risk of inflammation.

The fixtures are available in five different lengths (8, 9.5, 11, 14 and 17 mm) and three diameters (3.5, 4.5 and 5.5 mm). This system is also colour coded and hence allows easy recognition of the components that need to be used.

The fixture surface is the same acid-etched 'cell plus' surface used in the F2 and XiVe implants, thus reducing the integration period. Site preparation is undertaken in two stages: the machine-driven stage and manual preparation. The principles of drilling remain the same as with other systems, with adequate cooling and no overheating of the bone being prerequisites. The site is prepared with machine-driven instruments first and completed with two manual preparation steps using the conical reamer and the tap, both of which have non-cutting tips (see Fig. 3.49). The cover screw is pre-fitted onto the fixture and is only removed prior to threading in the abutment.

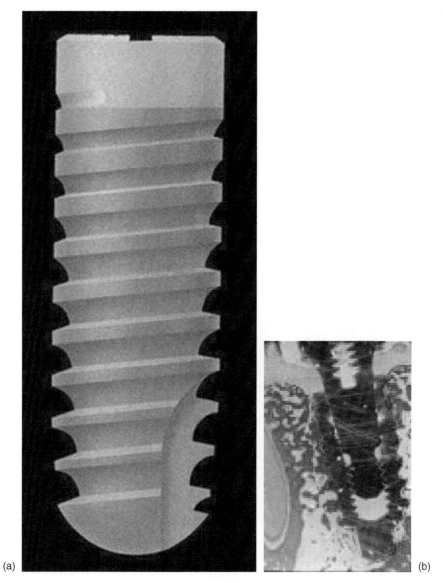

(a)

(b)

Figure 3.47 **(a)** The Ankylos implant. **(b)** The increased engagement of the apical threads into bone

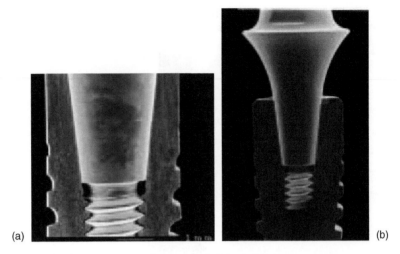

(a)   (b)

Figure 3.48 **(a, b)** The unique internal connection of the Ankylos system

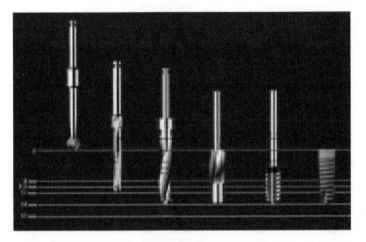

Figure 3.49 The drilling sequence. The last two drills, the conical reamer and the tap, are both hand-held and are the last step in site preparation prior to fixture placement

Prosthetic components

There are two main types of abutment: the balance base abutment and the syncone abutment. The latter is used when there is slight divergence of implants. In addition there are ball and socket abutments and also a syncone abutment for immediate loading. The geometry of the conical connector is identical for all implant diameters and abutment sizes, thus making the abutments freely interchangeable. The diameter of the abutment is determined by the diameter of the implant used. Fig. 3.50 shows the range of abutments available.

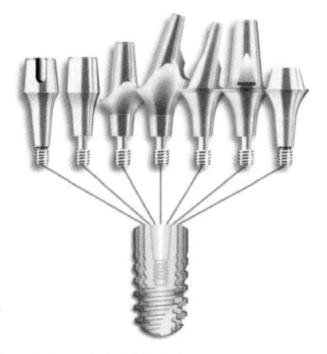

Figure 3.50 Range of abutments in the Ankylos implant system

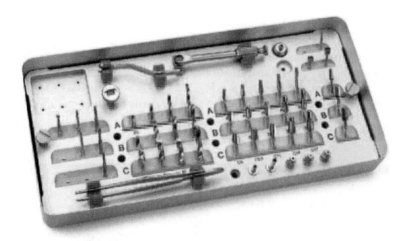

Figure 3.51 Ankylos surgical kit

Instrumentation

This system follows the same concepts as the XiVe surgical kit, with simplicity and colour coding being the key. Fig. 3.51 shows the surgical kit.

The 3i (Implant Innovations Inc.) System

The 3i (Implant Innovations Inc.) system is an American system and is owned by the Biomet Company. Originally marketed predominantly in the USA, the system has now gained acceptance throughout Europe, including the UK. The original design concepts were similar to those of the Brånemark System®, with some minor differences. The product line was marketed on simplicity and range. Although the natural taper(NT) implants are also marketed by the company, this chapter will only focus on the cylindrical implants. The design and concepts for the NT remain the same as the others, with the main difference being the use of tapered drills for site preparation.

Implants

Although originally the first implants were only available as external hex fixtures, these have been largely replaced by the use of the internal connection configuration called 'certain' implants. The range of fixtures available is vast and includes tapered implants (NT) and cylindrical implants. The certain implants are named as such due to the unique 'click' mechanism that is audible when the impression copings and abutments are seated onto the fixture. The system also offers expanded platform implants where the body of the implant has a smaller diameter with an expanded platform to facilitate an improved emergence profile for the restoration. This implant is designated the XP implant and is available in both external and internal configurations. Fig. 3.52 shows the range of fixtures available, and Fig. 3.53 shows the main differences between standard and XP fixtures.

The internal hex configuration has a click mechanism such that when the prosthetic components are seated an audible click is heard, confirming accurate seating of the component onto the implant (see Fig. 3.54) thus avoiding the need for taking verification radiographs. With the recent drive towards bone preservation, Biomet

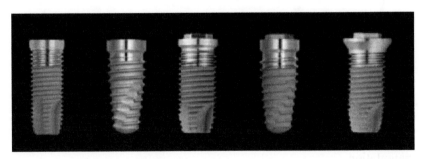

Figure 3.52 Range of fixtures available with the 3i system: the standard certain, NT certain, external hex standard, external hex NT and XP

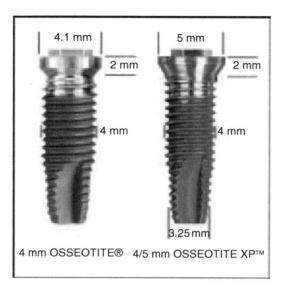

Figure 3.53 The difference between the standard fixture and the XP fixture

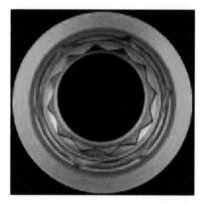

Figure 3.54 The internal connection of the 3i system

3i has introduced the 'prevail' implant, which is based on the philosophy of shifting the prosthetic microgap more medially on the implant platform, thus enabling bone preservation (see Fig. 3.55). Whilst this implant has been around for a while, the long-term outcome remains to be seen, although early reports appear promising. With all the different types of implants the apical cutting edge of the fixture is designed as an incremental cutting edge to facilitate self-tapping of the implant into the bone. The even distribution of the flutes ensures that maximum contact is maintained with the bone during the placement (see Fig. 3.56).

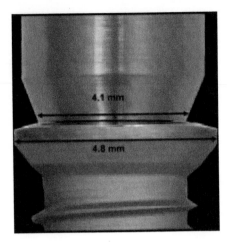

Figure 3.55 The prevail fixture with the microgap at the fixture abutment being shifted medially, thus preserving the bone

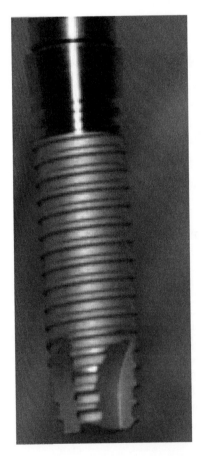

Figure 3.56 The incremental cutting edge design positioned apically on the hybrid osseotite surface

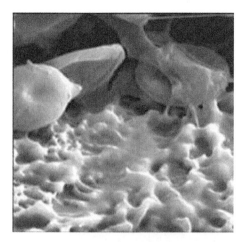

Figure 3.57 Electronmicrograph of the osseotite implant surface

The fixtures are available in six lengths (7, 8.5, 10, 11.5, 13 and 15 mm), with up to 20 mm available if needed, and four diameters (3.25 mm (micromini), 4.00 and 5.00 mm (standard) and 6 mm (wide)). With the external hex a diameter of 3.75 mm is also available. This does not include the XP platforms, which are available on the 4.00 and 5.00 mm fixtures as 4/5 and 5/6 mm.

The first implants were pure machined surfaces, but these have now been replaced by the osseotite surface. This is an acid-etched surface that enhances the rate of integration (see Fig. 3.57). The implants were originally marketed as a hybrid design with the coronal one-third of the implant being pure machined (see Fig. 3.56) to minimize bacterial colonization if the implant were to become exposed. However, this design is now being changed to a full osseotite surface where the etched surface reaches the top of the implant. The osseotite surface is currently being modified using nanotechnology to improve the integration rate and this implant is called the nanotite implant.

The drilling sequence follows the same stages as previously discussed with the other systems, with round and twist drills being used. However, when the XP implants are used an additional countersink is needed to flare the coronal aspect of the site to allow for the expanded platform. Fig. 3.58 shows the drilling sequence for the XP fixture. These implants do not need a mount and the driver for the certain implant has a unique configuration, as shown in Fig. 3.59. The driver has two markings, which enable the depth of insertion to be determined, for example subcrestal or at the crest.

Prosthetic components

The 3i System has a large family of preformed and custom abutments as well as the zirconium abutments. The gingival abutments are the most popular, with

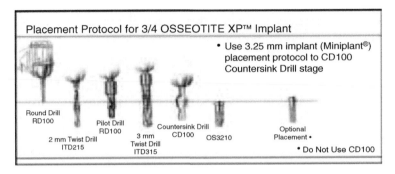

Figure 3.58   Drilling sequence for the XP fixture

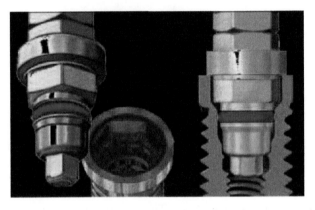

Figure 3.59   The fixture driver being inserted into the fixture for pick up prior to placement

the design of the abutments being the same for both the external and internal hex connections. Abutments are available for both cement and screw-retained prostheses. Figs 3.60a, b show the range of abutments available.

This system has a different healing abutment called the emergence profile abutment. It is designed to shape the gingival tissue following second-stage surgery to provide a shaped gingival collar prior to prosthetic replacement (see Fig. 3.61).

Instrumentation

The original surgical kits have now been replaced with simpler colour-coded kits, as shown in Fig. 3.62. The colour coding makes it easier for the assistant to follow thorough and match the drilling sequence to the implant. The prosthetic kit has a manual torque driver, and a smaller torque driver that only has a forward action with a 20 and 35 Ncm torque has also been introduced (see Figs 3.63a, b).

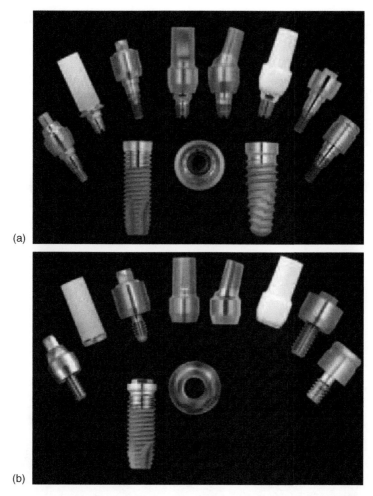

Figure 3.60 **(a)** The different abutments available for the internal connection. **(b)** The different abutments available for the external hex connection

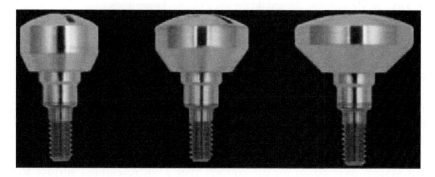

Figure 3.61 Emergence profile healing abutments

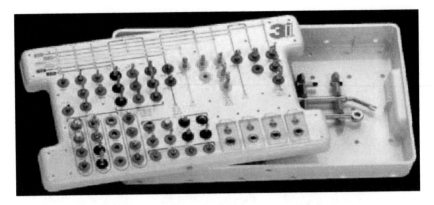

Figure 3.62 3i surgical kit

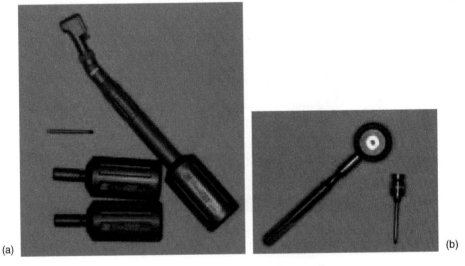

(a)

(b)

Figure 3.63 (a) The prosthetic kit and (b) the small manual torque driver

The Astra System

The Astra System was introduced to the market for clinical use in 1992. This system was based on the concepts postulated by Dr Stig Hansson and was one of the few systems at the time to have an internal conical joint compared to the external connection found in the majority of the systems. The unique features of this system were based on the concept that a microtextured surface to the top of the implant would help with bone preservation, the internal conical

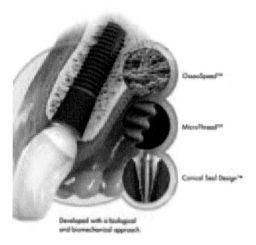

Figure 3.64 The design features of the Astra implant system

connection would help with more favourable load distribution, and microthreading to the top of the implant would help to improve load distribution but also retain crestal bone and the collar would help to reshape the connective gingival tissue. Hence this implant carried the four features of microtexturing to the top of the implant, internal cone, microthreading and the connective tissue contour (see Fig. 3.64).

Implants

The implants for this system are manufactured for use as a two-piece system. The implants have a unique design configuration with a roughened surface, microthread coronally and a conical connection of the implant to the abutment.

The original implant surfaces were created by means of a titanium oxide blasting procedure and the surface was called TiOblast. This surface now has been superseded by the osseospeed surface. This surface is a chemically active surface modified with fluoride to increase bone formation and enhance the bone to implant bond (see Figs 3.65a, b, c). The fixtures have a microthread coronally. These are minute threads that offer lower stress values and optimal stress distribution. This design is thought to promote bone preservation and maintain bone levels at the coronal aspect of the implant (see Figs 3.66a, b). The conical connection is called the conical seal design (see Figs 3.67a, b). This is a conical connection below the marginal bone level and it imparts load transfer deeper into the bone. The deeper connection is thought to reduce the peak stresses during function, thus enabling preservation of the marginal bone. Additionally the connection design seals off the interior of the implant from the surrounding tissues by moving the microgap away from the bone and increasing

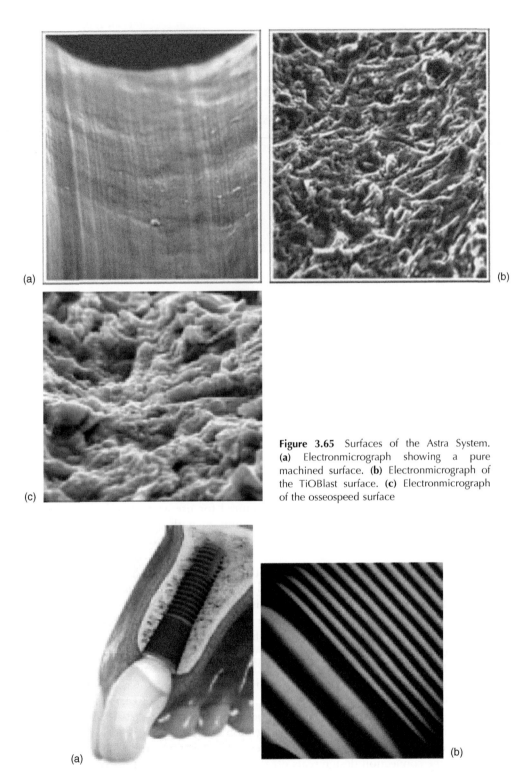

Figure 3.65 Surfaces of the Astra System.
(a) Electronmicrograph showing a pure machined surface. **(b)** Electronmicrograph of the TiOBlast surface. **(c)** Electronmicrograph of the osseospeed surface

Figure 3.66 **(a)** The coronal microthread configurations of the Astra System. **(b)** The electronmicrograph shows the threads closely

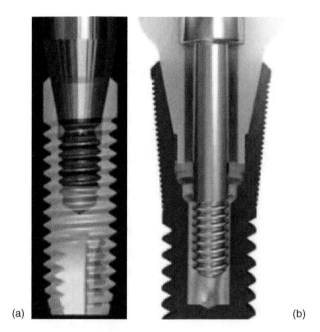

(a)　　　　　　　　　　　　　　　(b)

Figure 3.67 **(a, b)** The unique conical internal connection

the connective contour, thus reducing any microleakage and minimizing micro-movements. The precision fit of the connection makes the fitting of the implant to the abutment a simple procedure.

The implants for this system were manufactured as a straight/conical design, with the coronal third as the conical shape. Today a new fixture called the 5.0 straight is also available. The entire fixture from the neck to the apex is 5.0 mm wide. This implant has been designed for use in sites where improved primary stability is needed and it has all the same design features as the conical implant (see Figs 3.68a, b).

The conical implants are available in two different diameters, 4.5 and 5.0 mm, and the straight implants are available in three diameters, 3.5, 4.0 and 5.0 mm (see Fig. 3.69). The 3.5 mm and 4.0 mm straight implants are available in lengths of 8, 9, 11, 13, 15, 17 and 19 mm, with the other diameters available in lengths of 9, 11, 13, 15, 17 and 19 mm (see Figs 3.70a, b).

The drilling sequence remains the same as for previous systems and follows a series of sequential steps with a range of drills being used (see Fig. 3.71). In this system the countersink is called the cortical drill and for the conical fixtures there is also a conical drill (see Fig. 3.72).

Prosthetic components

The prosthetic components for both types of implants remain the same as the connection is the same. The healing abutments come in various sizes (see

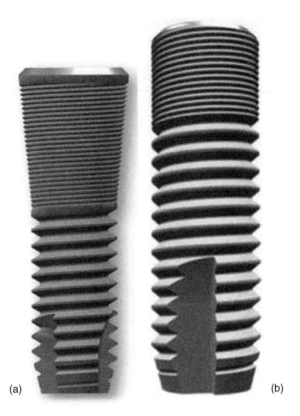

(a)   (b)

Figure 3.68 **(a)** The conical design of the Astra System. **(b)** The straight design compared to the conical design

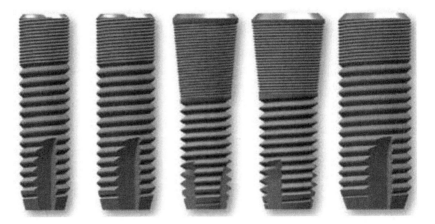

Figure 3.69 Different diameters of the system in the conical and straight fixtures

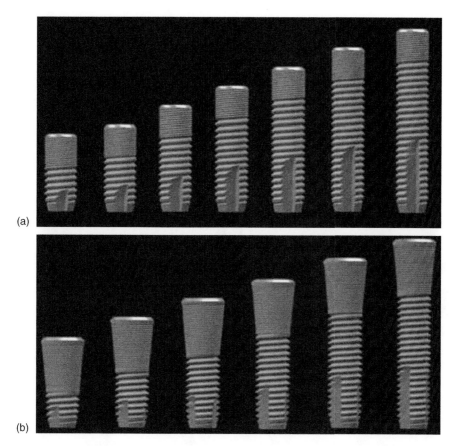

Figure 3.70 (a, b) The range of fixture lengths and diameters available. The 5.00 mm straight is also available up to 19 mm but this is not shown in this figure

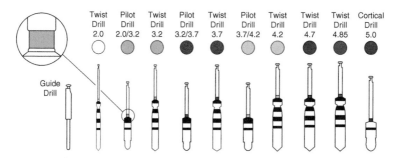

Figure 3.71 The range of drills. All the drills are colour coded. The last drill is the pilot drill. There is a cortical drill, which is the equivalent of the countersink

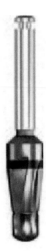

Figure 3.72   The conical drill used to prepare the conical flare for conical fixtures

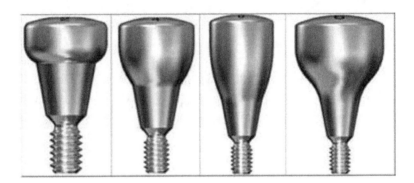

Figure 3.73   Range of healing abutments

Fig. 3.73) and the conical shape apically allows for the contouring of the gingival tissues during second-stage healing. The main difference with this system is that when the abutment is connected to the implant, a unique contour is created, as shown in Fig. 3.74, which allows for increased soft tissue contact both in height and volume, and closer integration into the transmucosal part of the implant, thereby sealing off and protecting the marginal bone. As with other systems there are both preformed or custom abutments available. Angled abutments are also available. As with the other systems, there is also a zirconium abutment available. Fig. 3.75 shows the range of prosthetic abutments available. This system also has a direct abutment.

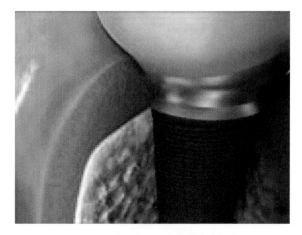

Figure 3.74   The connective tissue contour when the abutment is connected to the implant

Instrumentation

The surgical tray is compact with clear marking showing the assistant the drilling sequence and components needed (see Fig. 3.76). The prosthetic kit is compact and has a manual torque driver (see Figs 3.77 a, b).

Choice of implant system

The choice of system will usually be determined by the clinician and will normally be driven by the case mix and type of patients attending the clinic for tooth replacement with dental implants. The patient's need is determined by clinical assessment and the choice of system will be dependant on the needs of the patient groups seen and also the clinician's skills and familiarity with a specific system. Over and above the need for evidence-based outcomes, familiarity with the system selected will remain the key factor in ensuring predictable outcomes at a local level. The majority of the systems on the market today have developed products offering a wide range of choices both for fixture placement and restoration, but the following parameters should be taken into account when choosing a system:

- a proven track record of success
- should have strong implants and ideally must be made of commercially pure titanium or a titanium alloy that does not compromise osseointegration
- should have versatile prosthetic products and offer the option of being used as a one-stage or a two-stage system
- should be user friendly and easy to follow and learn.

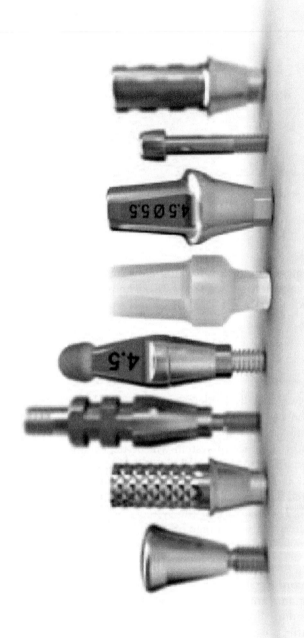

Figure 3.75 Range of abutments available for the Astra implant system

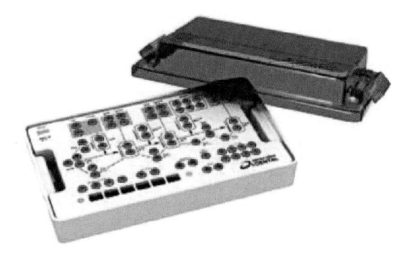

Figure 3.76 Surgical kit for the Astra System

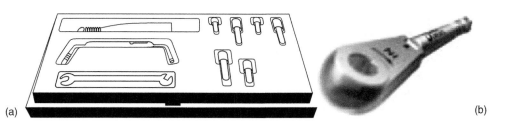

(a)   (b)

Figure 3.77 **(a)** Prosthetic kit with **(b)** the manual torque driver

Irrespective of the system used, it is important to be familiar with the product range and components to ensure that the procedure, once started, goes smoothly. Most companies will offer training courses for nurses and clinicians as well as chair-side support as and when necessary. The need for regular updates is also crucial to ensure that product knowledge and changes in the product range are kept updated, especially as all the companies regularly update existing products or introduce new ranges within their product line. This is especially important for dental nurses, who will be expected to set the procedure up for all the three stages: surgical, prosthetic and follow-up. To ensure that the products are maintained and serviced, on completion of the surgical procedure the components used during surgery, especially the drills, must be carefully disinfected and decontaminated. This is a stepwise procedure that is covered in Chapter 8. The onus for this falls onto the nurse and hence it is important that the nurse's product knowledge and decontamination protocol are up to date. Additionally, the nurse will need to record and log the number of uses of each drill for the multiple-use drills and reorder these as needed.

Conclusion

This chapter details the different implant systems. However, it is clear that the concept and methodology of all the systems remains the same and each of the companies have now resorted to simplifying their equipment and kits with colour coding. Most systems adopt colour coding to simplify the sequence of procedures, thus making the procedure much more user friendly. The nurse's role in the field of implantology cannot be underestimated. Nurses need to be familiar with systems and products to ensure that the correct procedures are followed in relation to site preparation and prosthetic connection as well as disinfection, and that the correct products are available on the day of treatment. Invariably the nurse will have to deal with the companies in ordering products and components for the treatment as well as when there is a problem and the only way this can be achieved is by ensuring that their product knowledge is up to date.

Surgical overview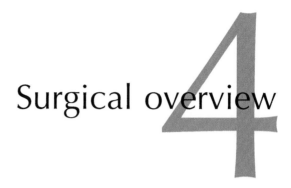

There are two main prerequisites for successful implant treatment:

- well-performed preoperative examination
- well-performed pretreatment planning.

Although this chapter focuses on surgical intervention to place dental implants, the importance of the above two parameters cannot be underestimated and their role in achieving the optimum outcome for the patient must be appreciated.

The surgical phase of implant treatment involves all the procedures that are necessary to get the fixture into or onto the jaw bone to facilitate the prosthetic phase. Whilst the surgical placement of dental implants is only one of a sequence of events that leads to an implant-retained restoration, it is a critical part of the overall sequence as the successful outcome is dependant on having the fixture successfully retained in the jaw bone. Prior to the surgical placement being undertaken it is crucial that the patient has undergone a comprehensive planning sequence to help ascertain their expectations against the limitations posed by the clinical environment in the patient's mouth as well as assessing the need for grafting and the appropriate type of surgical intervention.

Preoperative examination

The preoperative planning includes a decision-making process that helps to identify the level of the patient's compliance, motivation and dental awareness. This phase normally starts with identifying the patient's concerns, which are addressed by taking a good history from the patient, including details of why the teeth were lost and over what period of time. Additionally, details about the presenting concerns should also be taken and what outcome the patient is seeking. A careful medical and dental history is also undertaken during this phase.

The examination itself will include an extra-oral assessment followed by an intra-oral assessment. During the former factors such as facial asymmetry, the patient's smile line and any other abnormal features are identified. The clinical examination is undertaken in a systematic manner with an assessment of the soft tissues, the periodontium (this includes oral hygiene evaluation, gingival health and probing depths), the teeth (state of the teeth – restored or unrestored, any drifting or overeruption and position), the occlusion (both in intercuspal and retruded positions) and the existing prosthesis if one is worn. The examination should also assess the site of the missing teeth, the amount of space present and the gingival tissues in relation to the space. Once this is completed radiographs are taken, which may include a dental pantomogram (DPT) or periapical (PA) views.

At the end of this preoperative assessment, an indication of the patient's suitability for implant treatment should have been obtained. A differential diagnosis with a prognosis of the remaining teeth is made and finally an initial treatment plan is drawn up. During this plan any primary disease or abnormal findings should be addressed prior to the pretreatment planning phase for the implant treatment. Teeth with a questionable to poor prognosis are identified during this phase and a plan to either retain or extract them is made depending on the impact on planning. Teeth which are deemed to compromise the implant treatment should be considered for extraction, with a clear explanation to the patient of why this is being done.

Pretreatment planning

All treatment involving the replacement of missing teeth should begin with planning at the tooth level. This means that the final and intended position of the replacement teeth must be determined first before the surgical placement of the implant is planned. This position is usually determined with a diagnostic wax-up (discussed later) (see Fig. 4.1). The wax-up is used to transfer the tooth position by means of a guide to the radiographic assessment and the surgical placement. The surgical placement of the implant should be determined by a prosthetically driven treatment plan which enables an assessment to be made of the quantity of bone present in the site being considered for implant placement and the need for bone grafting either prior to the fixture placement or at the time of placement. This prosthetically driven plan will also enable the surgeon to ensure the correct fixture position in relation to the restoration and the limitations that may be encountered during surgery.

Whilst prosthetically driven planning is of paramount importance, it is also important to judge and plan the patient's suitability to undergo implant

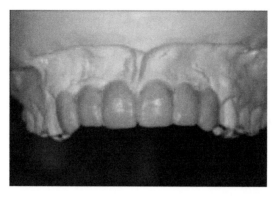

Figure 4.1 Clinical picture showing missing teeth and the diagnostic wax-up used to determine the intended position of the replacement teeth

treatment, which invariably involves a surgical procedure. It is crucial that prior to any planning for replacing missing teeth with dental implants the following has been achieved at the end of the preoperative examination and planning phase:

- active pathology in the oral tissues has been treated, for example denture-induced stomatitis or anaemia
- there is no complicating medical history
- primary disease such as caries, periodontal disease and teeth with hopeless prognosis has been dealt with.

Once the stability of the oral tissues and teeth has been achieved and the plan has been made to undertake replacement of the missing teeth with dental implants, the planning usually proceeds with further assessment of the patient's needs and expectations. These needs may have changed over the course of the preoperative treatment and it is important that these issues are clarified again to ensure that the patient's wishes are met. Once this has been accomplished, the site-related evaluation can take place. This is normally undertaken at two levels, surgical assessment and surgical planning, with surgical intervention only being undertaken after these have been completed.

Surgical assessment

During this assessment the patient's suitability to undergo surgery is ascertained. In particular their medical history is checked. Whilst there are no absolute contraindications to implant treatment, a number of conditions can affect the surgical intervention with compromised healing and reduced success. The medical conditions that should be carefully considered are endocrine disorders such as uncontrolled diabetes mellitus, uncontrolled granulomatous diseases and those with haematologic disorders such as haemophilia, who have increased risk of bleeding. The patient's smoking history is also crucial as heavy smokers have been shown to have a higher failure rate with dental implants.

During this phase other aspects that need to be assessed are the patient's ability to tolerate long surgical procedures in the dental chair and also the intra-oral opening of the mouth. Limited mouth opening can pose problems of poor access for instrumentation, especially at the back of the mouth. If all these factors are deemed favourable, then surgical planning is undertaken.

Surgical planning

Surgical planning involves the site-specific assessment of the area in which the implants are to be placed. During this phase, the proximity of local anatomical factors needs to be considered. These should be assessed in relation to the site of placement. The key anatomical structures that are important are:

- maxilla: position of the maxillary sinuses, the incisive canal and the nasopalatine foramen; the nasal cavity and the location of the palatine vessels and the root position of the teeth adjacent to the site of fixture placement
- mandible: position of the inferior dental canal in relation to the alveolar crest, the mental foramen and the genial tubercles, and the root proximity of the teeth adjacent to the site of implant placement.

A safe distance of at least 2 mm is needed between the anatomical structure and the implant (see Fig. 4.2). At this stage a judgement of the interarch and interdental spaces needs to be made. The smallest interdental space that can be accepted is 7 mm. This can be assisted with the use of a guide constructed from the diagnostic wax-up. Specific surgical planning is undertaken only after the

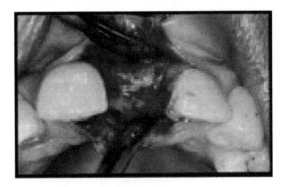

Figure 4.2   The proximity of the incisive canal to the site of fixture placement. At least 2 mm of clearance is required

above has been evaluated and must involve an assessment of:

- soft tissues
- hard tissues
- type of implant placement.

Soft tissue assessment

The quality of the gingival tissue biotype, for example is it thin or thick, is assessed and the presence of any muscle attachments which may affect the handling of the flap are also evaluated (see Figs 4.3a, b). If the site of implant placement is in the aesthetic zone, the smile line should be assessed and the relationship of this to the gingival margin examined (see Fig. 4.4). Whilst it remains a debatable issue, the presence of keratinized tissue and the need for soft tissue grafting either prior to fixture placement or after fixture placement should also be addressed at this time.

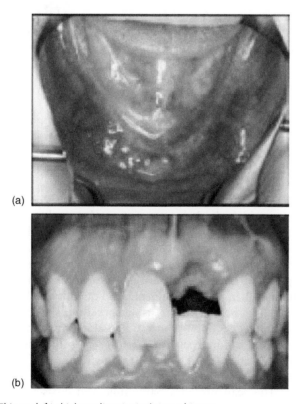

(a)

(b)

Figure 4.3 (a) Thin and (b) thick quality gingival tissue biotype

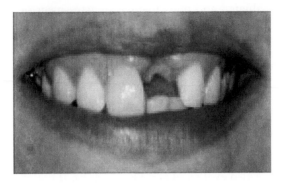

Figure 4.4   A high smile line with missing tooth

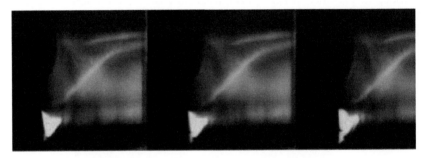

Figure 4.5   Lateral tomogram showing the outline of the tooth position (opaque outline of tooth) in relation to the underlying bone

Hard tissue assessment

The hard tissue assessment involves checking the position of the teeth in relation to the underlying bone (see Fig. 4.5). The tooth position is determined using the diagnostic wax-up, which also helps to ascertain the number of teeth that are to be replaced. The latter is important as this will help with deciding on the number of fixtures needed to replace the missing teeth. The bone quantity and quality are generally determined by the use of radiographs. The quality of bone, discussed in Chapter 2, will help to determine the choice of implant to be used and also the timing of implant placement. The quantity of bone, for example volume and height, can be determined using special radiographs, such as lateral tomograms or computerized tomograms (CT). Lateral tomograms can be advantageous to use as they are inexpensive, but they do sometimes have the disadvantage of being difficult to read. With CTs, the accuracy of the data obtained is improved and a computer program reconstructs data from a series of axial CT scans. The scan provides panoramic and cross-sectional views (see Figs 4.6a, b).

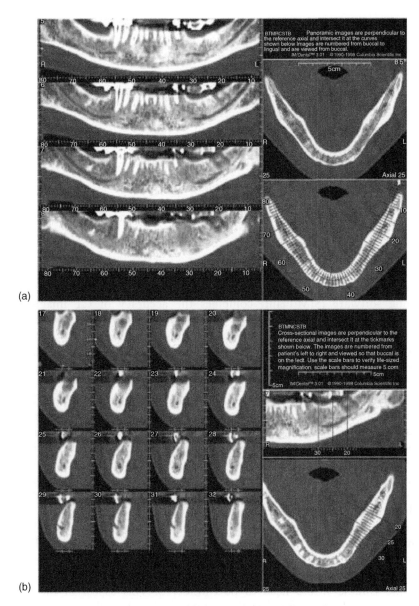

Figure 4.6 Computerized tomogram showing **(a)** panaromic and **(b)** axial views

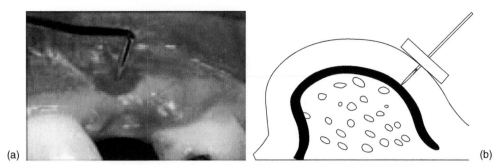

(a)   (b)

Figure 4.7 (a, b) Sectional stone cast showing the outline of bone obtained using bone sounding

The use of interactive CT data was introduced in 1993 and the preoperative planning software (SIM/Plant) combines the accuracy of CT imaging with the power of computer-aided design (see Chapter 6). This development has led to improved planning in difficult cases and surgiguides can be constructed using the information obtained. These can be used during the surgical placement of the fixtures. The information obtained from these special radiographs can be enhanced by the patient wearing a radio-opaque radiographic stent constructed from the diagnostic wax-up, which will show up on the radiograph. However, if these facilities are not available then bone sounding can be undertaken to assess the volume of bone present. Bone sounding requires local anaesthesia in the potential implant site and the depth of soft tissue is recorded at intervals along the proposed implant site. This information is transferred to a stone cast of the site which has been sectioned in the same alignment at which the measurements were taken. The readings are then joined to give an outline of the bone width (see Figs 4.7a, b).

The minimum bone volume required for placing an implant is 7–9 mm in height and 4–6 mm in width for a standard implant of 3.75–4 mm diameter. These dimensions will change slightly if smaller or larger diameter fixtures are used. If these dimensions are not present then augmentation to increase the bone volume would need to be considered. This aspect of the surgical planning is vital to ensure that the fixture is placed in the correct position in relation to the underlying bone to achieve an aesthetic result. Bone augmentation, if needed, can be undertaken at different stages depending on the volume of bone missing. In cases where adequate bone is present to provide primary stability of the implant when placed in the jaw bone, augmentation if necessary can be undertaken at the time of surgical placement of the fixture. However, if the bone volume is deemed inadequate then augmentation is undertaken first to recreate the bone volume prior to the surgical placement of the fixture.

Type of implant placement

With advances in implant systems and surface topography, the traditional concept of extracting the tooth and allowing for healing prior to implant placement has now become almost extinct. There are different ways in which implants are now placed in the jaw bone following tooth loss:

■ Immediate placement: the implant is placed at the same time as the tooth is extracted. This option is not appropriate if the extracted tooth is infected. Although this option was popular a few years ago, the problem associated with bone resorption during the immediate postoperative healing period has led to this method of placement becoming unpopular. This type of placement needs a higher level of planning and understanding of the healing response to avoid any aesthetic problems later on. If primary stability of the implant is not possible to achieve, then immediate placement cannot be undertaken (see Figs 4.8a, b).

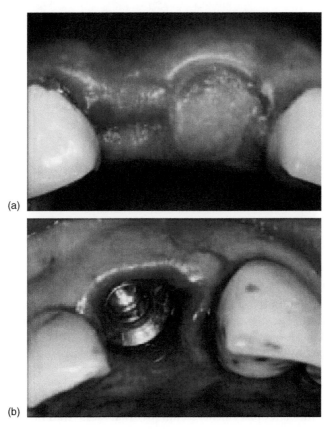

(a)

(b)

Figure 4.8 **(a, b)** Extraction of root and immediate placement of the fixture. At least 1 mm of bone needs to be present circumferentially if this option is to give a predictable outcome

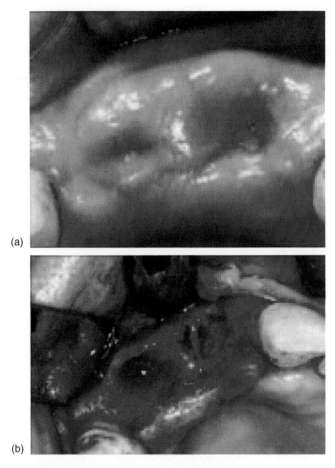

(a)

(b)

Figure 4.9 **(a, b)** Delayed placement. The extraction socket is allowed to heal for a period of 6 weeks during which time the soft tissues heal prior to placement of the fixture

■ Delayed placement: the tooth is extracted and the gingivae are allowed to heal. The implant surgery is undertaken 6 weeks after the extraction. The 6-week healing period allows soft tissue healing and minimizes the risk of unpredictable post-extraction bone resorption. For predictable outcomes, it is crucial that the implant has good primary stability when placed in the jaw bone (see Figs 4.9a, b). This is the most common type of surgical placement that is undertaken today.

■ Standard placement: the tooth is extracted and the site is allowed to heal for a period of 6 months before the implant surgery is undertaken. This is the late placement technique that was traditionally used (see Figs 4.10a, b).

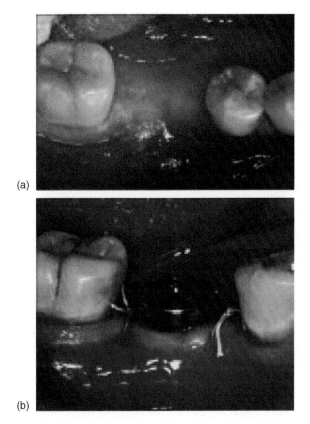

(a)

(b)

Figure 4.10 **(a, b)** Standard placement where the fixture is placed at least 6 months after the extraction of the tooth

Surgical placement

The main aim of surgical placement is to provide the anchorage for the planned prosthetic reconstruction. It is important to remember that the jaw bone into which the fixture is screwed is living tissue and as such needs to be handled carefully during the surgical procedure. The surgical protocol must be closely adhered to and all surgery must be performed according to the defined guidelines. These guidelines are generally the same for all systems but there are some small subtle differences. Details of the surgical protocol for implant placement are covered in Chapter 6, but this chapter focuses on the other surgical parameters that are also important. The nurse will need to ensure that the surgical set-up and appropriate instrumentation is available and in working order, including all the materials needed for augmentation and suturing. The surgical set-up is undertaken using a sterile aseptic technique, which is covered in Chapter 8. It is normal to use two clean nurses and one dirty nurse during the surgical placement. However, where this is not possible the nurse will need to communicate with the clinician on the best way of setting up the surgical instruments. In these situations the clinician will normally handle the drills. The surgical placement needs to be considered in three parts: the flap, the site preparation and the fixture placement. The surgical intervention should be undertaken using an aseptic technique with optimum sterility to reduce the risk of contamination and infection.

Types of flap

Two different flap designs were originally advocated: vestibular (made in the sulcus) or crestal (in the middle of the ridge) incision. However, since implants have been used in partially dentate patients, flap designs have changed and are driven usually by the procedures that are to be undertaken during implant placement, for example whether augmentation is to be undertaken at the time of placement or not. The basic principles of flap design remain the same in that the flap should be broad based to ensure a good blood supply and should be designed to provide good access to the surgical site. With the increasing demand in aesthetics, papillary preservation flaps have been commonly used. Irrespective of the type of flap design, full thickness flaps are raised and it is important that all the periosteum is raised with the flap. The flap should be extended to beyond the mucobuccal fold, especially if there is a buccal concavity present. In sites where there are anatomical structures, for example mental nerves, the flap should be raised such that the anatomical structure can be clearly identified and protected. Once the flap is raised the site should be cleared of all soft tissue to avoid this getting caught into the drills. Fig. 4.11 shows a full thickness flap with a slightly palatal placed incision.

Site preparation

Once the flap has been raised the site is prepared for implant placement. Any irregularities on the bone are smoothed. The most important aspect of this stage is the continuous cooling of the bone during the preparation. If the bone is exposed to adverse frictional heat, the bone dies, causing problems with integration of the implant. The drilling technique used is a sequence of preparation steps with intermittent drilling, using copious irrigation with saline to allow regular cooling of the bone. When the bone is extremely dense the use of a screw tap is recommended. The drills used have depth markings and these should be checked to ensure that the correct drilling depth is met. It is crucial that the drilling sequence recommended by the manufacturers is closely followed to ensure that the site preparation is undertaken correctly to provide a stable implant. In situations where the bone is very soft (type IV) the site can be pre-

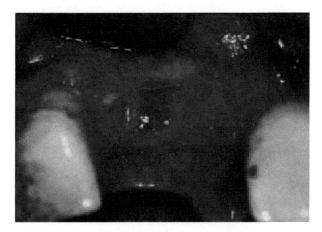

Figure 4.11   Full thickness flap exposing the site for fixture placement. Note the palatal position of the incision

pared using osteotomes (see Fig. 4.12). These are hand-held instruments with the same diameter as the drill that are used to expand the preparation site gradually to allow good stability of the implant once it is placed. It is normal to perforate the cortical plate with the round drill and the first twist drill to the required depth. The next sequence is then followed using the osteotomes to widen the socket to the required diameter and depth. Bone condensers have also been used for the same purpose (see Fig. 4.13) but unlike the osteotomes these do not have an apical cutting edge. The position and alignment of the implant site preparation is crucial to ensure that the implant is placed in the correct orientation for an aesthetic restoration. Normally the inter-implant distance (from the centre of one implant to the centre of another) should be no less than 7 mm, but 1 mm variation is accepted when smaller or larger diameter implants are used. The distance from the centre of the fixture to the adjacent tooth is usually around 3.5–4 mm. To achieve the required position of implant placement, a surgical guide should be used to ensure that the site of preparation is consistent with the required implant position. The size and length of implants to be used should have been selected in the presurgical planning phase.

Fixture placement and postoperative review

Once the site has been prepared the fixture is installed using machine-driven (handpiece) or hand-held instrumentation. The choice is usually dependant on the operator. Cooling of the fixtures during placement is no longer undertaken as this washes away the blood clot. Providing the site has been carefully prepared the implant should be firm and stable in its final position. This stability is referred

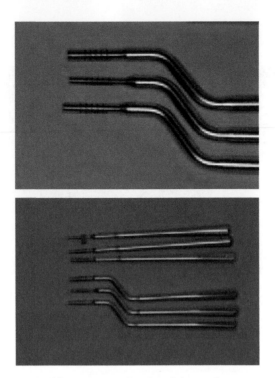

Figure 4.12 Osteotomes used for site preparation in soft bone. These osteotomes have an apical end cutting edge and can also be used for sinus elevation

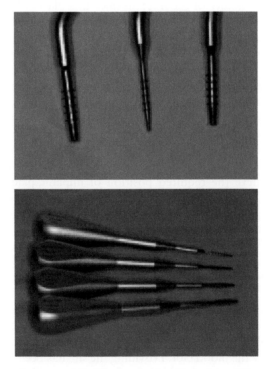

Figure 4.13 Bone condensers used for ridge condensing. These have a blunt end apically

to as primary stability and is essential to ensure a successful outcome. Depending on the type of placement, the implant is then protected with either a cover screw or a healing abutment. A cover screw is normally used when the implant is to be submerged under the flap. In these cases a second surgical procedure is needed to expose the implant and a healing abutment is then connected to allow for the gingivae to heal. The normal postoperative instructions for swelling, i.e. use of an ice pack to minimize the swelling and pain, are given. Patients are reassured about postoperative bleeding and the feeling of postoperative numbness, and difficulties they may encounter with speech and swallowing. Due to difficulties with cleaning, the patient is advised to use chlorhexidine mouth rinses for at least 1 week postsurgically. They are advised that they should not wear their removable prosthesis afterwards to avoid any untoward loading on the healing implants. Normally the patient will be reviewed 1 week later and at this time a radiograph should be taken to show the bone levels around the implant and the position of it. The prosthesis is adjusted and relined with a tissue conditioner at this visit. Future review visits are organized depending on the type of procedure undertaken and may be at 1 month and 3 months prior to the prosthetic phase starting.

Bone augmentation

Bone augmentation is used to try and re-establish the required bone width and height to facilitate fixture placement. Different types of bone augmentation techniques are used and can be undertaken either prior to the placement of the fixture (staged augmentation) or at the time of fixture placement (simultaneous augmentation). The advantage for the latter is that it requires minimum time and a reduced number of surgical treatments. However, the implant must have primary stability when placed. The former is undertaken when there is inadequate bone volume to place the fixture and achieve primary stability. In this situation, bone grafting is undertaken first and the graft is allowed to heal for a period of 6–8 months depending on the material used prior to reassessment for the surgical planning of the fixture. The planning of the bone augmentation procedures is undertaken at the same time as the surgical planning for fixture placement. A subsidiary planning approach for the specific augmentation procedures that are to be used should be undertaken to ensure that the risks, benefits and potential pitfalls of undertaking such procedures are evaluated.

Materials used for augmentation

A number of different materials have been used for bone grafting:

- Autogenous bone: this is bone tissue transplanted from one site to another in the same individual. This could be taken from a site in the mouth or from

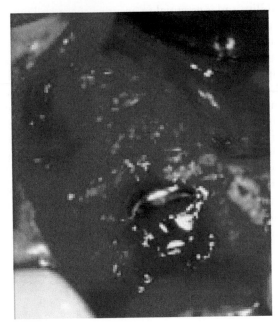

Figure 4.14   Autogenous bone used for grafting at the time of fixture placement. The bone was collected in the bone trap during site preparation

an extra-oral site such as the hip. The site from which the graft is taken is called the donor site and that into which it is placed is the recipient site (see Fig. 4.14).

■ Allogenic bone: this is bone tissue from the same type of individual. It is usually obtained from cadavers and the material is treated to eliminate any risk of infection by freeze drying, irradiation or acid washing.

■ Xenogenic bone: this is bone tissue from a different species, for example bovine (cow) bone. The most commonly used material in this group is 'Bioss' (see Figs 4.15a–c).

■ Alloplastic material: this is a synthetically derived material that does not have a human or animal source. Materials that fall into this category are the hydroxyapatites, bioactive glasses and calcium phosphate cements (see Figs 4.16a–d)

Although autogenous bone grafts give the best success rates, they require a second surgical site and the amount of bone collected is often inadequate. As a result of this alternative materials have been used, as described above. Autogenous bone grafts can be used as block grafts or particulate grafts where the bone is crushed into smaller particles. Different types of grafting techniques have been used and include grafts where a block of bone is placed on top of the underlying

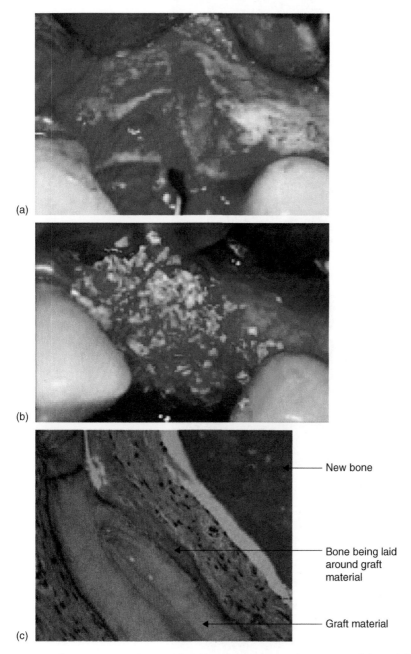

New bone

Bone being laid
around graft
material

Graft material

Figure 4.15   (**a, b**) Xenogenic graft material used to augment an extraction site with buccal dehiscence. (**c**) The histological picture shows some bone formation with some residual particles of graft material (light pink)

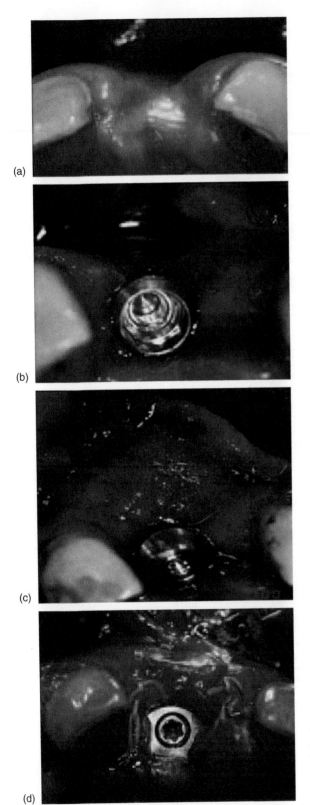

Figure 4.16 **(a, b, c, d)** Site augmented during fixture placement using a synthetic grafting material (bioactive glass). Note the change in the ridge contour that is achieved post grafting at 1 week review (d)

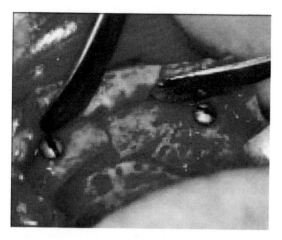

Figure 4.17 An onlay graft to increase the bone width for fixture placement

bone to increase bone volume (see Fig. 4.17) and inlay grafts where the bone graft is interspersed between two layers of bone to increase the height and/or width of bone. The particulate forms of grafting are used when bone augmentation is undertaken at the same time as the placement of the fixture.

Ridge expansion

This technique, also known as ridge splitting, is not exactly a bone augmentation technique but has been included in this chapter as it is used for restoring the bone volume in ridges that are very narrow. The thin bony ridges are split and widened to increase volume, with a grafting material inserted into the expanded area. The technique involves making an incision crestally on the ridge and a series of instruments called ridge expanders with increasing diameter are used to mechanically expand the ridge in the site chosen for the fixture placement. The ridge expanders are placed in position and gradually tapped with a mallet (surgical hammer). The expansion occurs by compression of the cancellous bone and pushing out of the cortical bone. Once the expansion has been achieved the implant can be placed into the expanded ridge and grafted with bone at the time of expansion, or the site grafted first and allowed to heal prior to the fixture placement.

Sinus floor augmentation

This procedure is undertaken in the posterior maxilla when there is inadequate bone height to place the implants, especially in the molar regions. This procedure is not suitable in patients who have sinus pathology, for example chronic sinusitis, those with excessive interarch distance, those in whom there are root tips left in the sinus and those who are systemically compromised. The maxillary sinus is the largest paranasal sinus and its anatomy must be closely studied if sinus augmentation is going to be undertaken. Maxillary sinus covers the roots of the teeth and is covered by periosteum. This lining is referred to as the schneiderian membrane. Sinus augmentation can be undertaken using two techniques and the choice of technique is based on the amount of residual bone present. Simultaneous augmentation is undertaken when there is a minimum of 5 mm of bone height. When there is little bone then a staged approached is undertaken so that the bone volume is re-established first before implant placement. This will add to the treatment time and it may take up to 9 months for the bone volume to be re-established. The sinus augmentation is undertaken either as a closed procedure, called an internal sinus lift (osteotome technique), or as an open procedure, called an external sinus lift (also known as the window technique). The osteotome technique is used when there is at least 4–5 mm bone height present and the sinus is approached via the site prepared for implant placement. The site to place the implant is drilled short of the sinus floor and sinus lift osteotomes are then used to carefully perforate the sinus floor and lift the sinus membrane up. Grafting material is pushed through the prepared site using the osteotomes to the required height in the sinus (see Fig. 4.18). The implant is then placed and the site closed. The window technique is used for direct access into the sinus and for the staged procedure where the grafting is carried out first. This is usually when there is less than 4 mm bone height. In this technique a window is prepared on the buccal aspect to gain direct access to the sinus floor, the sinus membrane is lifted and the graft placed into the sinus to

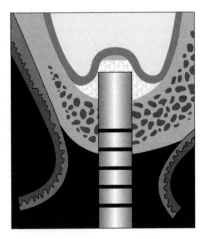

Figure 4.18 An internal sinus lift using osteotomes

the required height. The site is then allowed to heal prior to implant placement (see Fig. 4.19). The window technique can also be used for simultaneous placement of implants and the bone graft providing 5 mm bone is present and the fixtures are stable. Special sinus lift instruments are needed for the sinus lift window technique (see Fig. 4.20). Occasionally a tear can occur during the elevation of the membrane. If this occurs the extent of the tear is assessed and if it is extensive the procedure is stopped and site closed and allowed to heal. If the tear is small a resorbable membrane can be used to protect the tear. Clinically

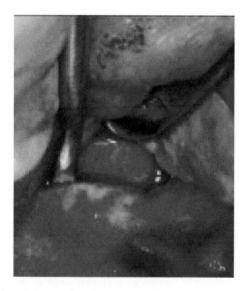

Figure 4.19   The window technique for sinus augmentation

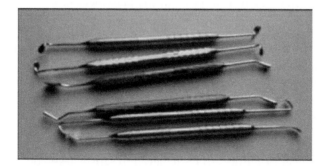

Figure 4.20   Set of sinus lift instruments

the clinician will pinch the patient's nose and ask them to blow gently. If bubbles are seen then the membrane has a perforation. Postoperatively the patient is given instructions for caring for the surgical area and specifically asked to avoid sneezing. In the event that there is a perforation, nasal decongestants can be prescribed. Implants placed in patients who have had sinus augmentation have been shown to have slightly lower success rates. The internal sinus lift procedure is now routine and has become an integral aspect of planning for patients to replace the posterior teeth with implants.

Guided bone regeneration

This is a technique that is used to reconstruct alveolar bone defects using a barrier. The barrier is used to create and protect a space for the blood clot to enable migration of the osteoprogenitor cells into the space, resulting in new bone formation. Today this barrier is used in conjunction with one of the grafting materials to enhance predictability. The barriers used initially were non-resorbable (called Goretex, made of expanded polytetrapolyethylene (ePTFE); see Fig. 4.21a) and had to be removed via a second surgical procedure following a period of healing which ranged from 6 to 9 months. Other non-resorbable materials used were the titanium mesh or shield which also had to be removed after 8–9 months depending on the type of graft material used (see Fig. 4.21b). To provide stiffness, gortex barriers were reinforced with titanium (see Fig. 4.22). These have largely been replaced by resorbable barriers due to problems of exposure and infection as well as the need for removal. Although synthetic barriers made from a combination of polyglycolic and polylactic acid are available (see Figs 4.23a, b), the collagen-based barriers are the most commonly used and are made either from pig (porcine) collagen or cow (bovine) collagen, each with slightly different handling properties. The porcine collagen barrier has a rough surface that faces the blood clot and a smooth surface that faces the soft tissues of the flap (see Figs 4.24a, b). The barrier can either be used as a simultaneous procedure during the time of implant placement or as a staged approach when the site is allowed to heal prior to the placement of the fixture at least 8 months later. The outcome is technique sensitive and the results can be variable. The main complication that occurs is exposure of the barrier, thus compromising the outcome. With the ePTFE barriers this was seen often, with infection being a common complication (see Fig. 4.25). In the event of this occurring the barrier had to be removed, thus compromising the healing of the regenerated tissue. However, with resorbable barriers this issue is not a significant concern as once the collagen membrane is exposed, early bioabsorption of the barrier is initiated. This may compromise the amount of bone regenerated, but to date this has not been of great concern. The technique of guided bone regeneration has enabled the ideal placement of fixtures to be achieved to satisfy aesthetic needs. As with all the other techniques, however, careful planning is essential to ensure predictable outcomes.

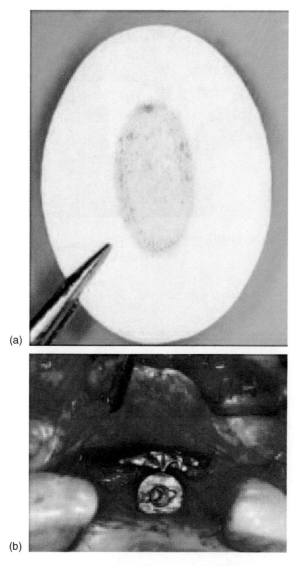

(a)

(b)

Figure 4.21 **(a)** A non-resorbable barrier (ePTFE) used for guided bone regeneration. **(b)** A titanium foil barrier in situ

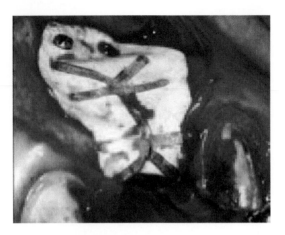

Figure 4.22   A titanium reinforced gortex barrier in situ

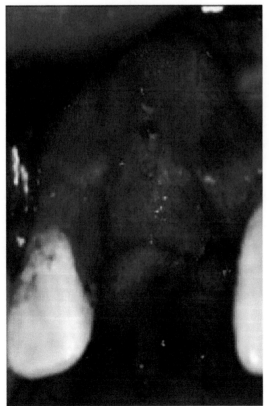

(a)

Figure 4.23 (a, b) A synthetic resorbable barrier in situ

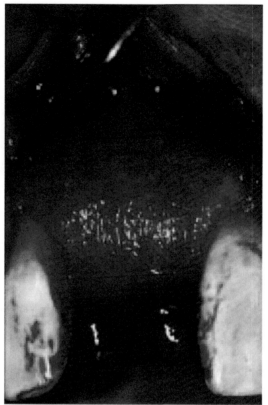

Figure 4.23 *Continued* (b)

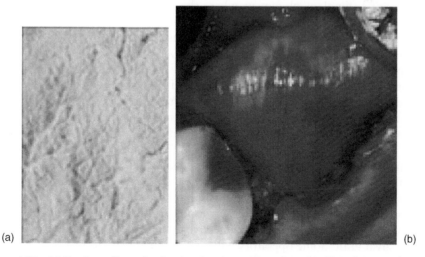

(a) (b)

Figure 4.24 **(a)** Porcine collagen barrier showing the rough surface. **(b)** Clinical picture showing the porcine barrier in situ with the shiny side facing the soft tissue

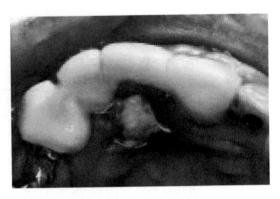

Figure 4.25   Exposed ePTFE barrier with infection

Soft tissue augmentation

The demand for enhanced aesthetics in treatment outcomes has resulted in a need for soft tissue grafting. The need for the presence of keratinized gingival tissue has been briefly touched upon, but despite the debate there are cases where soft tissues need augmentation to facilitate healing and aesthetic outcome of implant-retained restorations. There are two commonly used techniques for soft tissue grafting. These are the use of free gingival grafts to increase the band of keratinized tissue and the use of connective tissue grafts to increase the thickness of the tissues. The main advantage of the latter is that they offer a good colour match postsurgery to the augmented site. The grafting procedure can be undertaken prior to implant placement where the tissue quality is such that it may compromise the flap handling or at the time of first- or second-stage surgery or after the implant treatment where recession has occurred. Soft tissue grafting to date has usually been undertaken at second-stage surgery after the implant has been placed, but preoperative assessment and planning has highlighted a need for intervention much earlier. Figs 4.26a and b show a case which has been treated with a free gingival graft to augment the keratinized tissue width. The patient's presenting complaint of recurrent infections has been addressed following the placement of the graft. The free gingival graft is normally taken from the palate and placed at the recipient site. Figs 4.27a, b and c show a case in which a connective tissue graft has been used to enhance the gingival tissue thickness to eliminate problems with grey shine through the metal abutment. The connective tissue graft can be taken from the roof of the mouth via either a trap door incision, as seen in Figs 4.28a and b, or a pouch incision. The healing period is usually more comfortable with a connective tissue graft in the donor site than a free gingival graft. Some operators will use a healing plate to protect the donor site during the first few days following surgery. With a number of these proce-

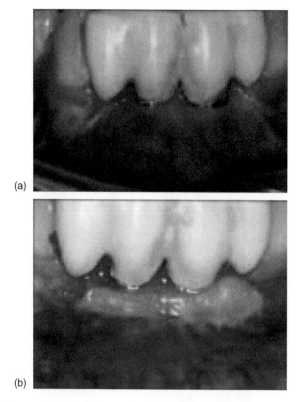

(a)

(b)

Figure 4.26 **(a)** Preoperative view of a case with dental implants showing the thin gingival tissue. **(b)** The same patient with a free gingival graft used to increase the keratinized tissue

dures smaller needle sizes of 5.0 or 6.0 diameter are used due to the nature of the gingival tissues.

With advancing techniques, the placement of implants in sites once deemed hopeless has become more predictable. However, this predictability relies on careful treatment planning and case assessment. Smoking does have a detrimental outcome on bone augmentation techniques and hence these procedures in smokers should be considered with caution. The surgical phase of the implant treatment is the most important phase. Although it forms part of a sequence of events, it is the most crucial step and requires careful thought and precision. Surgery that has been undertaken without due care and caution results in significant complications for patients and can in some situations render them worse off than when they started. Presurgical planning is essential to ensure that all potential complications have been addressed and identified to avoid any untoward problems.

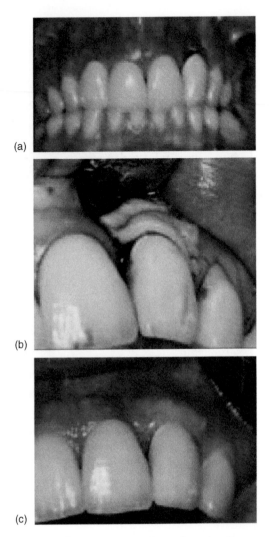

(a)

(b)

(c)

Figure 4.27   (a, b, c) Patient with a connective tissue graft used to increase the thickness of the gingival tissue following implant treatment where the grey metal of the abutment was shining through the thin tissue causing aesthetic concern. **(b)** The connective tissue graft with epithelial collar

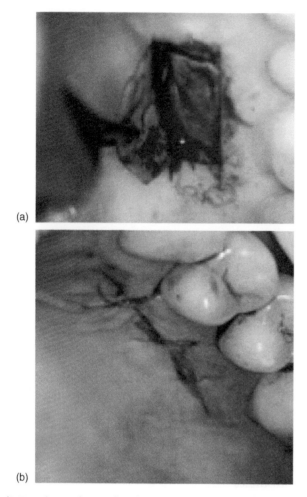

(a)

(b)

Figure 4.28   **(a, b)** Trap-door technique for taking a connective tissue graft. The trap door is sutured into place

Prosthetic overview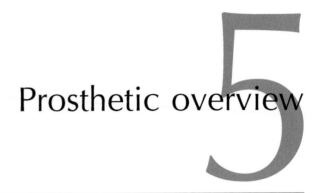

Patients with missing teeth do not like wearing a prosthesis that can be removed from the mouth. Previous chapters have provided an overview of the stages that are crucial in the construction of an implant-retained prosthesis. This chapter discusses the types of prostheses that can be constructed and the rationale for when the different types are considered.

There are three key groups of implant-retained restorations that need to be considered. These are:

- fixed prostheses
- removable prostheses
- fixed and removable prostheses.

Fixed prostheses

A fixed prosthesis is fixed to the dental implant and cannot be removed by the patient. This type of prosthesis can be a single tooth crown or multiple teeth. Most patients prefer to have this type of prosthesis as it closely resembles their own teeth. Multiple teeth can either be restored with a few implants which carry a number of teeth or retained on individual implants. The latter usually becomes costly due to the number of implants. Depending on the reasons for tooth loss, placement of multiple implants is not always possible due to inadequate bone volume and height. A fixed prosthesis usually replaces the missing teeth and only a limited amount of soft tissue can be replaced with such a prosthesis. The

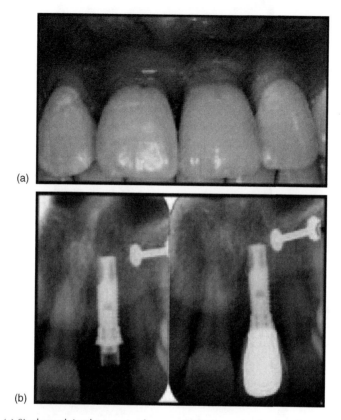

Figure 5.1 **(a)** Single tooth implant-retained crown. **(b)** Radiographs showing the ceraone abutment and the final crown in situ

decision to use a fixed prosthesis depends on the patient's expectations as well as the clinical situation in the mouth. The latter is assessed during the pre treatment planning phase and the suitability of a fixed prosthesis can be assessed depending on how much soft tissue has been lost and the impact of this on the patient's facial profile. Figures 5.1a, b and 5.2a, b show a single tooth and an implant-retained bridge replacing a number of missing teeth. The impact of replacing a denture with a fixed prosthesis on the patient's facial profile and lip support is seen in Figs 5.3a, b.

The fixed prosthesis can be retained either by screwing it into the implant or cementing it onto the abutment. A screw-retained prosthesis is easier to remove in the event of a problem and is screwed into the abutment with a prosthetic screw. Once the prosthesis is fitted, the crown will have an access screw hole through which the screw is accessed. This hole is then sealed off to protect the screw head. A screw-retained prosthesis is slightly more bulky than a cement-retained restoration (see Figs 5.4a, b). The torque used to screw the prosthetic

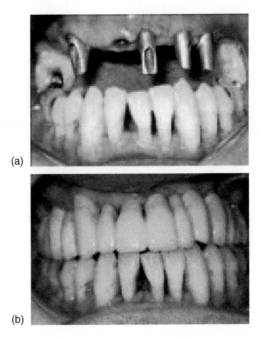

(a)

(b)

Figure 5.2 (a, b) Multiple missing anterior teeth replaced with a fixed implant retained reconstruction

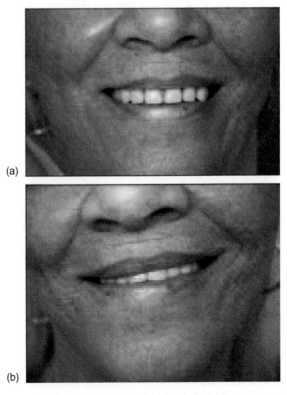

(a)

(b)

Figure 5.3 (a) Patient wearing an upper denture showing good lip support. **(b)** Same patient with the denture replaced with a fixed bridge. Note the loss of the labial lip support

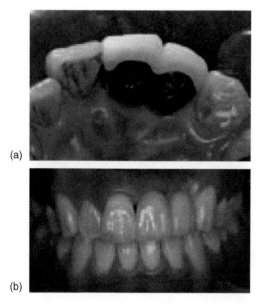

(a)

(b)

Figure 5.4 **(a)** Palatal view of implant support crowns that are screw retained. **(b)** Labial view of screw-retained crowns

screw is less than that required for the abutment screw. The clinician may periodically remove the screw-retained fixed prosthesis during the follow-up visit to assess the underlying implants and the soft tissue.

In contrast, a cement-retained prosthesis is cemented onto the abutment. When Temp Bond is used, retrievability is sometimes difficult. Today different manufacturers have introduced special cements for cementing implant-retained crowns. Cement-retained crowns are aesthetically more pleasing, especially in the front of the mouth (see Figs 5.5a–c).

Removable prostheses

A removable prosthesis is attached to the implants in a way that allows the patient to remove the prosthesis for cleaning. This type of prosthesis is retained by implants and is supported by the underlying soft tissue and bone. As a result the denture needs to be constructed using the basic denture principles. The implants offer retention for the prosthesis to help the patient function more effectively. The dentures can be retained on implants with either a stud-type attachment or a bar-retained attachment (see Figs 5.6a–d and 5.7a, b). Recently locator abutments have been used more often than stud attachments (see Fig. 5.8a, b). In the mandible a minimum of two implants are needed to retain a

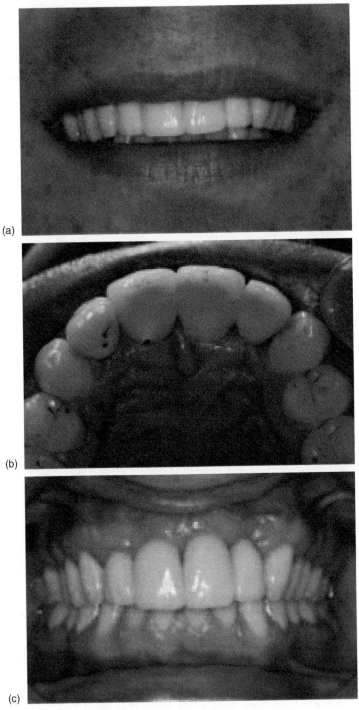

Figure 5.5   (a, b, c) Cement-retained crowns showing excellent aesthetics

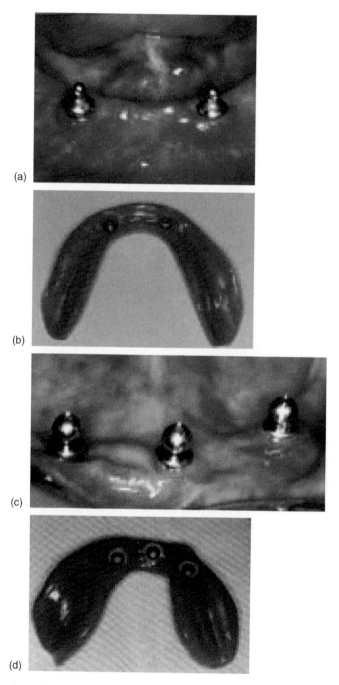

Figure 5.6 **(a, b)** Stud-retained lower denture on Straumann implants. Note the retaining clips in the denture. **(c, d)** Ball-retained lower denture on Brånemark implants. Note the 'o' rings in the denture

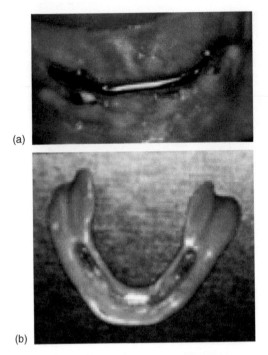

(a)

(b)

Figure 5.7   (a, b) Bar-retained lower denture. The clips retained in the denture attach onto the bar. Note that today the distal cantelevers seen are kept short

denture whereas in the maxilla a minimum of four implants are needed to retain a denture. The dentures are referred to as over-dentures. The abutment is connected to the implant and the denture houses either clips if retained on a bar or 'o' rings if retained on studs. With time these rings and clips may need replacement due to wear. This is a relatively simple procedure.

Although implant-retained dentures look exactly the same as conventional dentures, due to their improved retention they offer patients added security with function. A removable prosthesis also enables the restoration of lost soft tissue support and thus may in some cases offer better aesthetics than a fixed prosthesis.

Fixed–removable prostheses

This type of prosthesis is usually suitable in patients with full-mouth reconstructions. The fixed part is fitted to the implants and the removable part, the superstructure, (with the teeth), can be removed by the patient for cleaning. The superstructure fits over the metal part using friction. The minimum number of

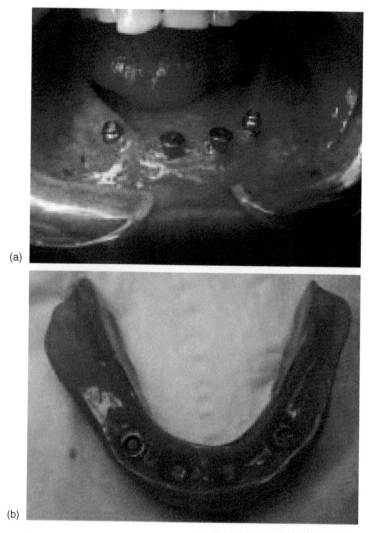

(a)

(b)

Figure 5.8 (**a, b**) Locator abutments in situ in a patient who has been rehabilitated following surgery for cancer. (**b**) Denture showing the keepers in situ

fixtures needed for such a prosthesis is five or six. The bar fixed to the implants is usually precision-milled. Figures 5.9 a, b show a milled bar used to retain a denture in a cleft patient.

Irrespective of the type of prosthesis, the sequence for construction of the prosthesis is the same. Once the implants have integrated, impressions are taken either of the implants or the abutments screwed into the implants. The different types of impression techniques have been covered in Chapter 2.

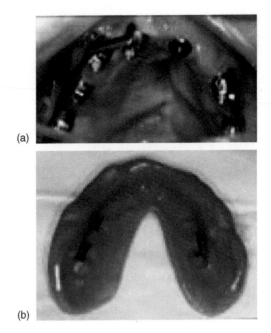

(a)

(b)

Figure 5.9 **(a, b)** Milled bar used to retain an upper denture in a patient with a repaired cleft

Traditionally implants were left to integrate into the jaw bone for 6 months, but with advancing technology and understanding, the impression can be taken:

- immediately at the time of placement during the surgical phase.
- 8 weeks after the surgical placement
- 6 months after the surgical placement.

Immediately at the time of placement

This type of impression can only be taken if there is adequate bone to support the implant and there is good primary stability of the implant. The impression is usually taken at the fixture level and sent to the laboratory. The laboratory then makes the restoration, which can be fitted onto the implant at the same visit. This option is not suitable if there is a lack of bone which has needed augmentation or the bone has been grafted.

Newer concepts of implant placement and reconstruction have also been reported by a number of implant companies and are referred to as 'implants in a day'. In these cases the implants are surgically placed and special tools are used to take impressions of the implants and the prosthesis is then connected to this.

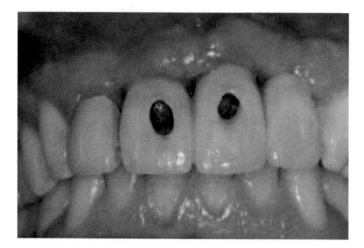

Figure 5.10 Temporary (also called provisional) crowns used to help guide the gingival tissues prior to the construction of the final crowns. The labial access holes are sealed with a tooth coloured material

8 weeks and 6 months after surgical placement

Impressions at this time are taken either at fixture level or at abutment level. With the latter the preformed abutment is connected to the implant, the impression taken and the abutment protected. Implants that have been placed as two-stage implants will need to have a second surgical procedure to expose the implants. The implants are connected to the mouth with healing caps. Today it is more common to place the implants in a one-stage procedure. Temporary crowns/restorations are usually constructed to allow the gingival tissues to mature prior to the construction of the final prosthesis. The temporary crowns are used to guide the gingival tissues to give the best aesthetic result (see Fig. 5.10).

Final impressions

The final impressions are taken after the tissues have matured (see Fig. 5.11). The nurse will need to ensure that the correct impression copings are ordered. A prosthetic kit with drivers will be needed and the special tray or adjusted stock tray made ready for the clinician. The impression material will need to be prepared and materials used for jaw registration also made ready. The impression coping is connected to the fixture or the abutment and the impression taken in addition-cured silicone material. The impression copings enable the fixture analogues to be connected such that the position of the fixtures in the mouth is

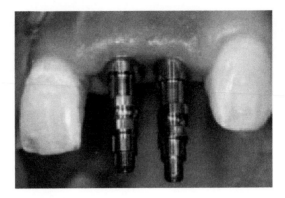

Figure 5.11   Fixture level impression copings

replicated on the stone model. The different types of prosthetic abutments have already been covered in Chapter 2 and vary depending on the system used. A shade is taken of the teeth and depending on the number of teeth missing either a jaw registration is taken or another appointment made to record the jaw registration using an occlusal rim. All the information is then sent to the laboratory technician, who will pour the impression and construct the crowns on either preformed or custom abutments if the impression is taken at fixture level (see later). As much information as possible, for example photographs, is sent to the technician to help in the construction of the prosthesis.

Laboratory stages of prosthetic construction

Once the impressions have been taken, they are washed and removed of all debris, blood and saliva, and disinfected prior to sending them to the laboratory. The nurse will need to ensure that the clinician has completed the required laboratory request form advising the technician of the type of prosthesis needed and what is required for the next phase. The nurse will usually collaborate with the laboratory for the date when the work is to be completed. Once the impression is received in the laboratory, the technician will locate the fixture or abutment analogues in the impression depending on the type of impression taken. The cast is then poured in improved stone, which is hard and does not break off. The models are then mounted on an articulator. The wax-up and stent should also be sent to the laboratory. The gold cylinders are then connected and depending on whether the prosthesis is a single or multiple unit, the hex or non-hex cylinders are used. The multiple units do not need a hexed cylinder as the framework will provide the anti-rotation need to secure the prosthesis in place. The prosthesis is then waxed to the required contour with waxing and laboratory screws. The wax prosthesis is cut back for the porcelain and the framework is cast. A polishing protector is used to protect the cylinder and abutment surfaces during the polishing. The fit of the prosthesis is ascertained and the porcelain is applied. The occlusion is checked and the prosthesis is finished and polished ready for insertion into the mouth. In cases with multiple teeth missing or where there is a high aesthetic demand, a framework try-in or biscuit bake try-in is undertaken to check the fit prior to the porcelain work being undertaken in the clinic.

Inserting the prosthesis

The whole assembly is returned to the clinic for fitting in the patient's mouth. The clinician will check the prosthesis outside the mouth first. The nurse needs to set up the surgery with the prosthetic kit and also ensure that the torque drivers are available. The prosthesis is tried in the mouth and the nurse will assist with passing the correct drivers and screws needed. This is especially important when multiple units are being fitted. The clinician may decide to take a verification radiograph prior to the final fit or cementation. The patient is shown the prosthesis and asked to make some speech sounds. If the patient is happy, the abutment is torqued to a predetermined value to the fixture. This step is important to prevent screw loosening in the future. Where there are multiple abutments, the laboratory constructs a jig to enable the correct orientation of the abutments to be achieved in the mouth (see Fig. 5.12). The restoration is then either cemented or screwed into the abutment. With the former, the access hole to the abutment screw in the abutment has to be sealed off prior to the crown being cemented (see Figs 5.13a, b). The occlusion is then checked and any minor adjustments undertaken, especially in lateral excursions. The clinician must ensure a passive fit of the abutments onto the fixture. This means that the abutment can be seated on the fixture without any force or pressure. The patient is

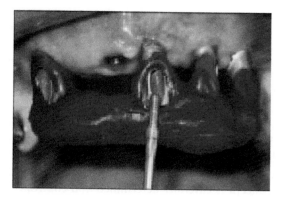

Figure 5.12 Duralay jig used to help screw the abutments to the fixtures in the mouth in the correct orientation

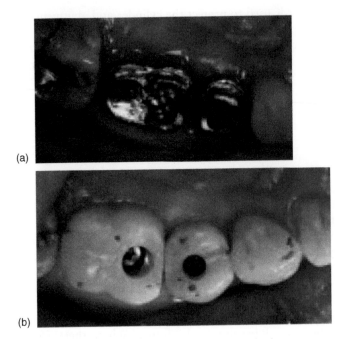

(a)

(b)

Figure 5.13 (a) Screw-retained framework connected in situ with abutment screws. (b) Screw-retained crowns showing the access hole, which will need to be sealed off

then sent home and a review appointment is arranged. A post-fit radiograph should be taken and this will then be used to assess bone level changes over time. Post operative instructions are also given at this visit.

Loading of the implants

Prior to advances in the topography of the fixture surfaces, the fixtures were traditionally not loaded until 6 months after placement. However, as surface configurations have improved, enhancing osseointegration, the concept of immediate loading has been introduced. This means that following placement the fixtures are loaded by constructing a prosthesis that enables patients to use the implant-retained teeth for function. Such concepts are used when 'implants in a day' are provided. It is important that this concept of immediate loading is not confused with immediate restoration, where the restoration is placed on the fixtures but is not loaded. This means that when the patient closes their teeth the implant-retained restoration is just out of the bite. The immediate loading concept does provide good results providing the patients are carefully selected and the loading concept is carefully determined and controlled. It is important, however, to remember that this concept is not suitable for the majority of patients.

Post-insertion instructions

Following the fit of the prosthesis, the patient should be advised on the care of their prosthesis. The nurse may play a role in offering this advice to patients and should therefore be aware of different ways of cleaning the prosthesis. The importance of thorough cleaning is emphasized and the patient shown how to access the prosthesis, especially on the fitting surface. Oral hygiene aides, such as superfloss, plastic-coated interproximal brushes and single-tufted brushes, should be recommended. Although the patient can use mouthwashes, an emphasis is placed on the role and importance of manual cleaning and the long-term use of chlorhexidene (corsodyl) discouraged. It is important that the patient is informed about the use of multiple aides to facilitate cleaning as usually no single aide is adequate. The cleaning is even more critical in patients with a history of periodontal disease. The efficacy of the cleaning should be monitored and assessed at every recall visit. This forms part of the overall care that the patient will need on completion of treatment.

The prosthetic phase of treatment is the final phase in the active course of treatment and gives excellent outcomes providing the cases are well selected and planned. The final outcome is determined by careful top-down or crown-down planning, which is critical to ensure that the patient has been made aware of the possible limitations well before the final prosthesis is delivered.

Indications for implant treatment and patient selection

Dental implants can be used to replace missing teeth, which often cause functional and social problems as a result of poor aesthetics. Tooth replacement therefore becomes necessary to maintain appearance, function and oral health by preventing drifting and tilting of teeth. Success rates of up to 95% have been quoted with dental implants. However, to ensure these high success rates good case selection and treatment planning are essential. The following factors should be taken into account when considering implants as a replacement option for missing teeth:

■ the cause of the tooth loss – this may affect the quality of the bone and soft tissue present.
■ the prognosis of the remaining dentition.
■ the impact of the replacement options on the remaining dentition and oral health.

It is important to remember that dental implants are an option for tooth replacement and other conventional methods of tooth replacement, such as dentures and bridges, should be considered when planning for the replacement of missing teeth. The main causes of tooth loss are:

■ *Periodontal disease*
Patients who have periodontal disease are not necessarily poor candidates for implant treatment. However, it is crucial that the periodontal disease in the rest of the mouth is treated and the prognosis of the remaining teeth considered. Implants in periodontally susceptible patients in whom the periodontal disease has been treated and stabilized with no recurrence have

been shown to have success rates that are slightly lower than in those patients with no periodontal disease. However, due to the extent of bone and tissue loss, these patients usually require some form of bone and soft tissue augmentation to facilitate implant treatment. These patients also need close monitoring to ensure that the periodontal disease remains stable and bone levels should be closely monitored around the implants and the teeth.

- *Dental caries*

  The caries risk for the individual must be identified as caries can ultimately lead to loss of remaining teeth, especially if there are large restorations in the mouth. It is important to contingency plan for future loss of teeth such that the placement of the implants does not compromise the alternative options should further teeth be lost.

- *Endodontic failure*

  Endodontic treatment usually gives good success rates over 10 years. However, problems related to poor coronal tooth tissue and root fracture need to be taken into consideration. The prognosis of endodontically treated teeth in the vicinity of the sites in which implants are to be placed need to be considered carefully to ensure that the implants have a predictable outcome.

- *Congenital absence*

  Patients who suffer from hypodontia are those who are born with some or all of their teeth missing. The teeth present are usually small (microdonts) and often are spaced unfavourably in relation to the missing teeth. In these patients the alveolar ridge in the area of the missing teeth is usually narrow with poor quality gingival tissue. These patients often need extensive treatment involving tooth movement with orthodontics to recreate the spaces. These patients, because of the poor quantity and quality of bone and gingival tissue, will need bone grafting to facilitate implant placement. Depending on the severity of the tooth loss, the more conventional forms of treatment may give better aesthetics and predictability.

- *Trauma*

  Teeth lost as a result of trauma often have additional soft and hard tissue loss. The type of trauma needs to be ascertained and the prognosis of the teeth determined. In some cases early loss of the tooth and replacement with a dental implant may provide a more favourable and predictable outcome by helping to preserve the bone.

Case selection and treatment planning

Once a decision to replace the missing or failing teeth with dental implants has been made, case assessment and planning are crucial to ensure an aesthetic and functional result. The following aspects should be ascertained during the preoperative and pretreatment planning phases:

- **Patient demand vs. expectations**
  The patient's demands against their expectations should be closely evaluated during the history taking. Patients with very high demands and expectations that are unrealistic may not be good candidates for implant treatment. The planning phase should take into consideration how realistic the patient's expectations are and whether implant treatment will meet these expectations. If there are any doubts then the alternatives to implants should be considered.

- **Medical history**
  Aspects of the medical history that contraindicate surgery should be looked at carefully as this may preclude the patient from having implants. Additionally, any factors that compromise the implant surgery or outcome need to be discussed with the patient and the risks involved explained. Patients with uncontrolled diabetes are poor candidates for implant therapy due to compromised wound healing. In these patients the diabetic status needs to be controlled first before any intervention is considered. Patients with atypical facial pain and depressive illness may not be good candidates for implant therapy.

- **Smoking history**
  Smoking is not an absolute contraindication to implant treatment but the success rates of implants in patients who smoke has been shown to be lower than in non-smokers. The patient should be made aware of this risk and advised to stop smoking at least 3 months before surgery for implant placement.

- **Dental history and experience of dental disease**
  This will help to ascertain the patient's attitude to dentistry, and their motivation and compliance towards dental treatment. A history of recurrent failing restorations should raise concerns about parafunctional (grinding) habits. These patients may have a poorer predictability for implant treatment due to excessive loading on the implant as a result of grinding. It is crucial that patients who grind (brux) and parafunction are identified as they may have a lower success rate with dental implants. Additionally, their occlusion may need to be assessed carefully during the planning phase.

Clinical examination

The clinical examination forms part of the pretreatment plan and should be carefully completed. The assessment should be undertaken in the following sequence:

- *General assessment*
  During the general assessment the smile line, periodontal status, restorative status, overall soft tissue health, occlusion and jaw relationship should be

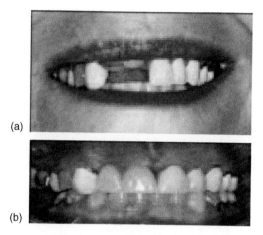

(a)

(b)

Figure 6.1 **(a)** The lips when the patient smiles. **(b)** The same patient with the denture in situ showing the need to carefully plan the replacement of the missing anterior teeth taking into consideration the future loss of the heavily restored remaining teeth

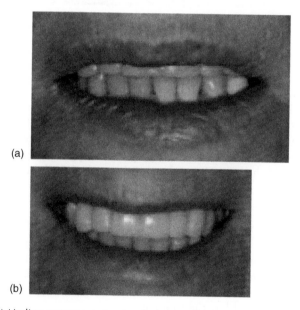

(a)

(b)

Figure 6.2 **(a, b)** Lip line assessment at rest and when smiling

given particular attention. In addition the value of the tooth to be replaced in the arch should be assessed as well as the periodontal and restorative predictability (see Figs 6.1a, b). These are aspects that need to be evaluated to ensure that the outcome to the implant treatment is not compromised. The patient's smile line needs to be ascertained and how much of the teeth they are showing at rest and when smiling (see Figs 6.2a, b).

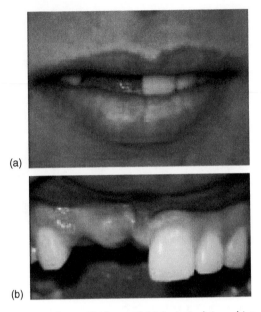

(a)

(b)

Figure 6.3   (a, b) Patient with a low smile line and thick gingival tissue biotype

- *Site-specific assessment*

    This should focus specifically on the site-related factors and include an assessment of the gingival soft tissue biotype (thick quality or thin quality), the morphology of the tooth/teeth to be replaced, and their relation to the adjacent teeth as well as the underlying bone support (see Figs 6.3a, b). The relationship of the opposing teeth and the occlusion should be checked (see Figs 6.4 a, b, c). The outline form of the ridge and the width should also be assessed (see Fig. 6.5).

- *Study casts and diagnostic wax-up* (see Figs 6.6 a–c)

    Articulated study casts are an invaluable tool for planning. They enable the sites to be examined from all sides and also give an indication of the amount of space available. The casts can be used to produce diagnostic wax-ups, which are replicas of the intended outcome of the final prosthesis. The wax-up is invaluable and has the following uses:

    - It can be used in the discussion with the patient, who can visualize what is proposed.
    - It can aid in determining the interocclusal and intraocclusal space available.
    - It can help in defining the shape and size of the tooth to be replaced. This information can also be used to help determine the size of the implants that would be needed for the restoration of the case.

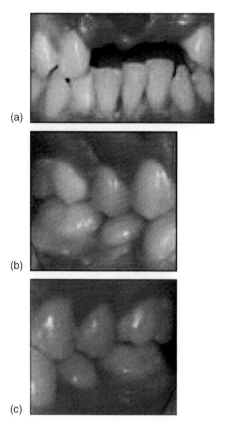

(a)

(b)

(c)

Figure 6.4 **(a, b, c)** Figures showing the missing teeth, the position of the frenum and the over-eruption of the opposing teeth anteriorly and good occlusal contacts posteriorly

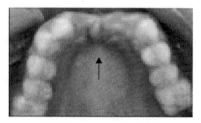

Figure 6.5 Palatal view showing the width of the ridge where the teeth are missing. Note the labial concavity and the anterior position of the incisive canal

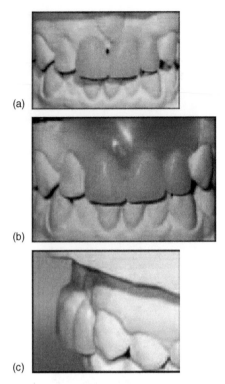

(a)

(b)

(c)

Figure 6.6 **(a, b)** Articulated study casts with the diagnostic wax-up of the teeth and the soft tissues showing tooth position and the soft tissue loss. **(c)** Side view of the wax-up of the teeth to be replaced

- It can be used to provide the radiographic template which the patient can wear when the radiographs are taken. The outline of the teeth to be replaced can be seen on the radiograph in relation to the bone volume.
- It can be used to make the surgical templates that can be used during surgery to ensure the ideal placement of the implant.

■ *Radiographic assessment*

The radiographic assessment is crucial to help ascertain the quantity and quality of bone present and the need for hard tissue augmentation. Standard radiographs such as dental pantograms (DPT) and long cone periapicals will only give a two-dimensional view of the area (see Figs 6.7a, b). Axial tomograms are also used to give an outline of the bone width. However these are still two-dimensional radiographs (see Figs 6.8a, b). In cases where there are anatomical difficulties or a close look at the anatomy is needed, three-dimensional views may become necessary. Computerized tomography (CT) scans (see Fig. 6.9) give a three-dimensional view of the teeth and the jaw bone as well as the anatomical structures. In the past few years, advances

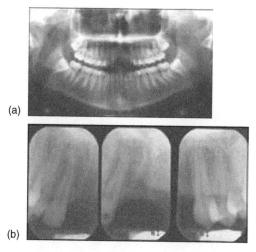

Figure 6.7 **(a)** Dental pantomograms of the same case. **(b)** Long cone periapical radiographs showing the prominent incisive canal

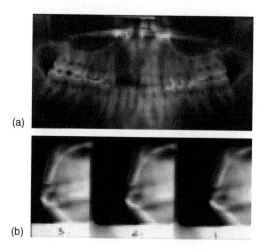

Figure 6.8 **(a, b)** The axial view magnified at 1.7 with the slices cut at a width of 4 mm showing the bone width

in computer technology have resulted in computer-guided implant planning (SIM plant) becoming popular for more complex and difficult cases (see Figs 6.10a–d). It is usual for the patient to wear a radiographic template to show the tooth position on the radiographs that are taken. In Figs 6.10b–d this is evident as purple teeth. The choice of radiographic assessment will depend on each case and needs to be balanced against the diagnostic value and exposure to the ionizing radiation. The radiographs are essential to help identify the presence of anatomical structures such as the inferior dental

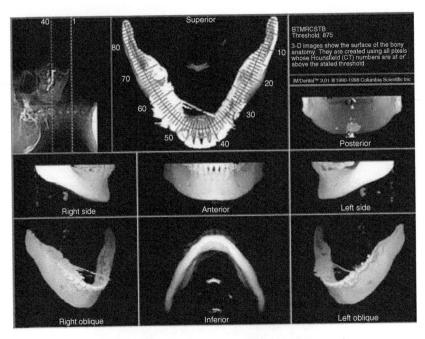

Figure 6.9 CT scan showing the bone contours and width from different angles

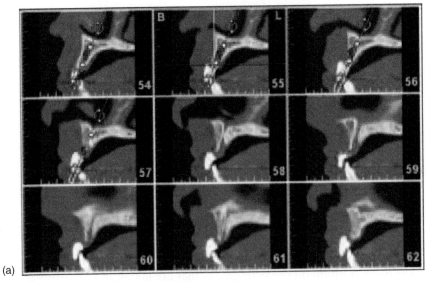

(a)

Figure 6.10 (a) CT scan with the SIM plant planner used for identifying the fixture positions in the jaw bone.

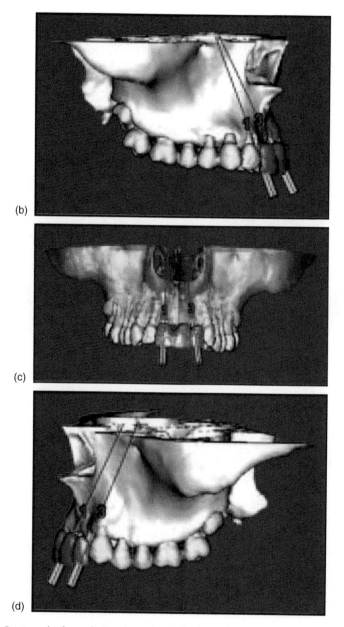

(b)

(c)

(d)

Figure 6.10 *Continued* **(b, c, d)** Simplant planner with tooth position shown in purple and the direction of the intended implant position

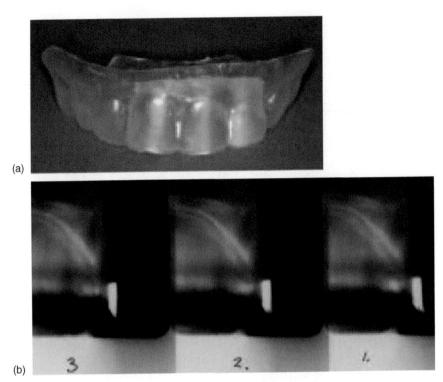

(a)

(b)

Figure 6.11 **(a)** Radiographic template with radio-opaque marker as seen on tomogram. **(b)** Sectional tomogram showing the marker identifying tooth position in relation to the underlying bone

canal, the incisive canal and the sinus in the relation to the site where the implant is to be placed.

- *Radiographic and surgical templates (also called guides)*
  Templates are used to show the position of the final prosthesis in relation to the underlying soft tissue and bone. Templates can be radiographic or surgical. The radiographic template has a radio-opaque material incorporated into it and the patient wears it before the radiograph is taken so that the outline of the final prosthesis is mapped on the radiographic image. This guide gives an indication as to the need for bone augmentation to facilitate implant placement in the desired location (see Figs 6.11a, b). The radiographic guide can also be subsequently converted to a surgical guide.

The surgical template provides the surgeon with a guide of where the final crown is likely to be so that the implant can be placed in the ideal position surgically. This template is made from acrylic or acetate and can have various surfaces cut away so that access holes can be drilled through it (see Fig. 6.12).

At the end of the case assessment and planning, the clinician should have a clear idea of the type of prosthesis needed, for example cement or screw-retained,

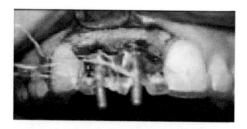

Figure 6.12 Surgical template in situ showing the access holes with the position guides verifying the site of fixture placement in relation to the crown of the tooth

and the need for grafting (bone and soft tissue) to place the implant in the prosthetically driven position. The diagnostic wax-up will also help to determine the number and size of the implants to be used, the type of surgical procedure to be undertaken and the overall treatment time from the placement of the implant to the fit of the crown.

The planning is also important to enable the clinician to consult the patient regarding the intended procedure, giving an indication of the potential risks associated with undertaking treatment with implants and the potential risk of failure. The patient must have been given all the alternative treatment options, including the implant option, so that they are able to make an informed choice of treatment. It is important to remember that implant surgery is a restoratively driven procedure.

Surgical procedure

Once the pretreatment planning is completed, surgery to place the implants can be undertaken. The planning phase pre-surgically will have provided a good knowledge of the surgical site and a surgical template can be used to help the placement of the implants in the correct position. The surgical placement of the fixture can be undertaken in one of two ways:

- *Two-stage procedure*
  The implant, once placed in the jaw bone, is completely covered over with gingival tissue. After an appropriate healing period the implant is uncovered with another minor surgical procedure (often called second surgery), exposing it in the mouth. This is a simpler procedure and is necessary to uncover a buried implant. It can be undertaken using a tissue 'punch' or by raising a flap. Depending on the tissue quality, a soft tissue graft (connective tissue) can be undertaken at the time of second surgery if needed. The cover screw is removed and a healing abutment is placed to connect the implant to the mouth (see Figs 6.13a, b and 6.14a, b).

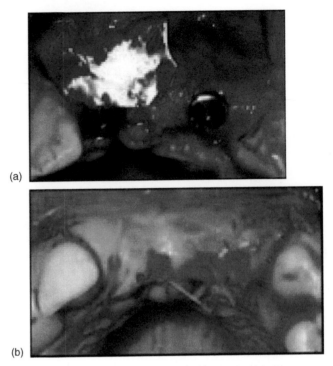

(a)

(b)

Figure 6.13   (a, b) Fixture placement with augmentation and closure following placement

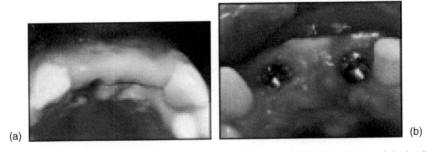

(a)   (b)

Figure 6.14   (a, b) Second stage surgery for the same case with a full thickness flap and the healing abutments in situ 1 week later

■   *One-stage procedure*

The implant, once placed in the jaw bone, is connected to the oral cavity using a healing abutment. This allows the gingival tissue to grow around it. Implants specifically designed to be used as one-stage procedures normally have a polished collar at the top of the implant, which allows the gingival tissue to grow round it. However, a number of implant systems designed for

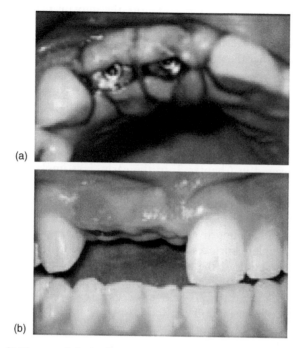

(a)

(b)

Figure 6.15 (a, b) The top of the healing caps are just visible at the end of the surgery, unlike Fig. 6.13b and also at review 1 week later.

two-stage use can be used as one-stage systems. The main advantages of the one-stage system are that it reduces the healing period before which the prosthetic phase can start, avoids the need for a second surgical procedure and allows uninterrupted healing of the gingival tissue around the implant (Figs 6.15a, b).

Implant surgery is an exacting procedure and needs to be undertaken with a degree of precise handling of both the soft tissue and bone. Any traumatic intervention will lead to complications and potential problems. The type of flap raised should be a full thickness flap and should give good access to the surgical site. As part of the site preparation, residual tags of granulation tissue are removed and irregular bone contours smoothed prior to starting the drilling sequence. The site preparation is carried out atraumatically using the standardized drills, starting with round drills followed by the twist drills with copious cooling. The site is sequentially prepared and gradually increased in size to the required diameter and length. Throughout the drilling sequence the position is verified using position indicators and the surgical guide. The final drill is usually slightly smaller that the implant itself. Most of the companies now provide self-tapping implants, which enable the implant to be placed into the prepared hole without pre-tapping. In situations where the bone quality is Type I/II (very hard bone), the site may need to be screw tapped before the implant placement so that the implant can be inserted without generating any heat or trauma to the site. It is crucial that there is no overheating of the bone during the drilling and placement. Depending on whether the procedure is one- or two-stage, either a healing abutment or a cover screw will be placed to protect the top of the implant before the gingival flap is replaced and sutured without any tension. Figures 6.16 a–l show the stages undertaken surgically to place two fixtures for replacing the missing anterior teeth.

The drilling sequence is similar for nearly all systems, but depending on the type of placement and the fixture there may be minor differences. These have already been covered in Chapter 3. In the early days implants were placed as 'late' implants, where once the tooth was lost the gingival tissue was allowed to heal for a period of at least 3–6 months before any planning for the implant surgery was undertaken. However, today more partially dentate patients are having implants and the improved and shorter times needed for osseointegration with the newer implant surfaces as well as the need for bone preservation, the time between extraction of the tooth and placement of the implant have been reduced significantly with implant placement now undertaken either immediately (at the same time as extraction) or 6–8 weeks later after the soft tissues have healed. Standard placement still continues to have a role in those patients who lost their teeth many years ago.

The healing abutments used at first- or second-stage surgery are available in different configurations depending on the system used. The height of the healing abutment is determined by the thickness of the gingival tissue. Following a healing period of 4–6 weeks, depending on whether soft tissue surgery has been undertaken or not, the patient is ready for the prosthetic part of the treatment.

Prosthodontic procedures

The prosthodontic procedures on dental implants follow similar principles to those of conventional crown and bridgework. The final outcome and success is dependent on the position of the implant in the jaw bone in relation to the final restoration. Once the healing period for the integration is complete, the process for the construction of the prosthesis starts. The type of restoration to be placed should have been decided at the planning stage. The choice of the abutment to be used is determined by the implant angulation and position, the gingival height, the aesthetics and the space present.

The prosthodontic phase starts with taking impressions of the implants in the jaw bone. The details of the different impression techniques have already been covered in Chapter 2.

If the impression is taken at implant level, the impression copings are connected to the implant and the impression taken. If a decision has been taken to use a machined (preformed) abutment, then this is connected to the implant with

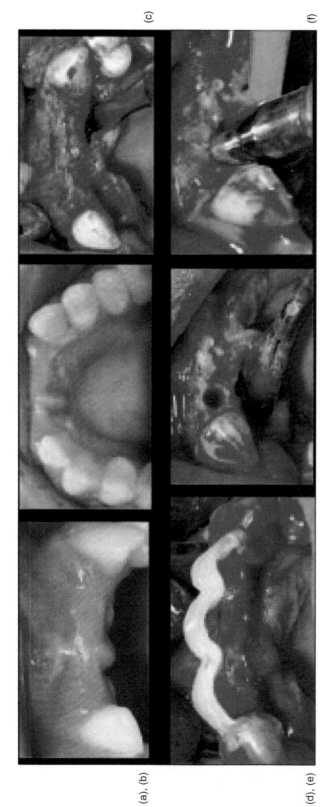

(c)

(f)

(a), (b)

(d), (e)

Figure 6.16 (a) Preoperative labial view of patient with missing anterior teeth. (b) Palatal view of the same patient. (c) Full thickness flap raised to expose the underlying bone. (d) The surgical template in situ. (e) Site prepared with the first twist drill using the guide. (f) Fixture being placed in prepared site.

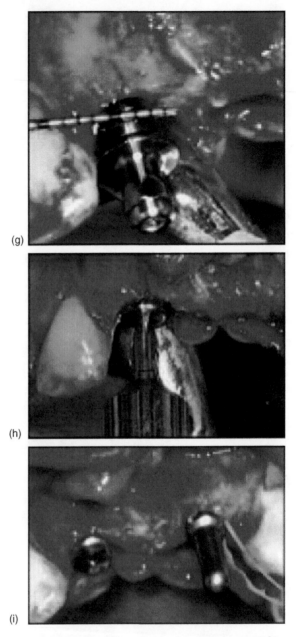

(g)

(h)

(i)

Figure 6.16 *Continued*   **(g)** Verification of the position of the fixture. Note the fixture mount. **(h)** The mount has been removed and the cover screw placed to protect the fixture head. **(i)** The second site being prepared. The position indicator (alignment pin) in situ helps to guide the site preparation in relation to the position of the first fixture.

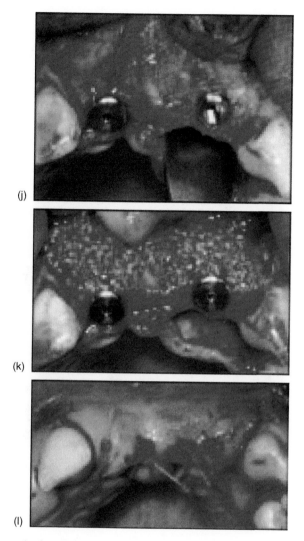

Figure 6.16 *Continued*   **(j)** Both fixtures in site. The left fixture does not have the healing cap (cover screw). **(k)** Labial augmentation at the time of surgery using bovine bone. The fixtures had good primary stability and are protected with the healing caps. **(l)** Flap replaced with both fixtures buried under the gingivae

the abutment screw and torqued to the required level. The torque is necessary to provide the preload on the abutment screw to prevent screw loosening when the prosthesis is fitted. The shoulder of the abutment needs to be kept at least 2 mm below the gingival margin to maintain aesthetics. The impression coping for the abutment is then seated and the impression taken (see Figs 6.17a–c). The abutment needs to be protected when connected in the mouth (see Fig. 6.17d). Verification radiographs are sometimes taken when the impression coping or

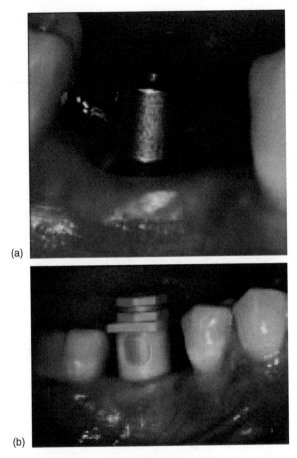

(a)

(b)

Figure 6.17   (a) Solid abutment of the Straumann system connected in the patient's mouth to the fixture. (b) White plastic basket and positioning cylinder in situ to take the abutment level impression.

abutment is connected to the implant to ensure that the coping or abutment is seated down on the implant platform and there is no gap. When implant level impressions are taken the transfer caps or impression coping are connected to the implant, as shown in Figs 6.18a–c.

Once the impression has been taken, a facebow record is taken if necessary. A jaw registration is taken to ensure the correct occlusal relationship, but if there are enough teeth present to locate the casts in intercuspal position then a registration is not always necessary. A shade of the teeth is taken. The impressions, jaw registration and shade are sent to the laboratory with a written prescription. The laboratory connects the analogue to the impression and pours this up into a cast. The abutment is then connected to the implant and the provisional or definitive restoration constructed.

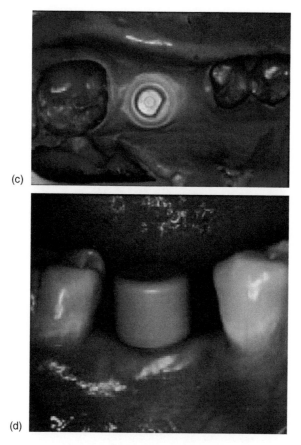

Figure 6.17 *Continued*   **(c)** Impression showing the abutment level impression coping picked up in the impression. **(d)** Solid abutment protected with a temporary cap

The cast with the restoration is then delivered to the clinic for trying the prosthesis into the patient's mouth. If the try-in is satisfactory, the restoration is either screwed or cemented onto the abutment. If an implant level impression was taken, a locating jig is used to connect the abutment in the mouth to ensure the correct alignment into which the crown fits. If the crown is cemented then usually temp bond is used. Alternatively special cements for implant-retained restorations can be used. Figures 6.19a, b show the clinical case with the fixtures and abutments connected in the mouth. Figure 6.19c shows the verification radiograph once the abutments are connected. Figures 6.20a, b show the definitive crowns cemented in place with the final radiographs. For screw-retained restorations, the access hole is sealed off as a temporary measure. The choice between the two will depend on the need for retrievability and the aesthetic demand. The main advantages of a screw-retained prosthesis are that it is easily retrievable but occasionally the screws can become loose, indicating functional

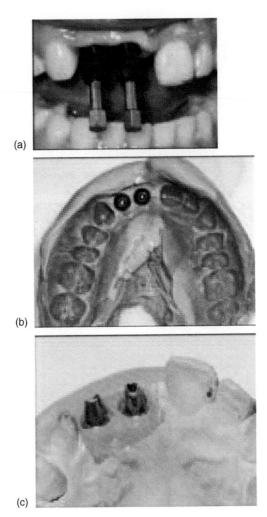

(a)

(b)

(c)

Figure 6.18 **(a)** Fixture level impression copings in situ for an open-tray impression techinque. The screws will project out of the impression tray. **(b)** Impression taken in addition-cured silicone with the impression copings in situ. **(c)** Laboratory stone cast poured up with custom abutments onto which the crowns are made

overload, and the prosthesis can also be bulky. In comparison, the cement-retained prosthesis may provide better aesthetics but retrievability maybe difficult and excess cement can be extruded into the soft tissues. The occlusion is also checked.

Follow-up care

Once the implant-retained restorations are fitted, the patient should be reviewed at least 2 weeks later to assess how they are getting on. If all is satisfactory then

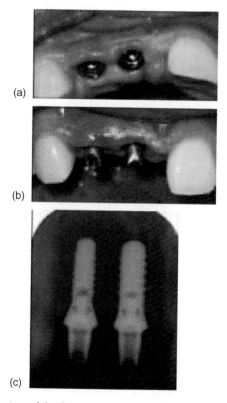

Figure 6.19 (a) Clinical view of the fixtures in the mouth following removal of the healing caps. (b) The abutments connected to the fixture and torqued. (c) Verification perapical radiographs showing the seating of the abutments

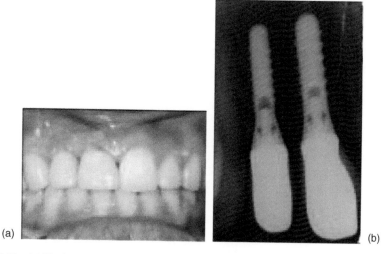

Figure 6.20 (a) Final crown cemented in place. (b) Radiograph taken following cementation of the crowns. This will be used to assess the bone levels during recall

the patient is placed on annual recall. It is important that radiographs are taken when the prosthesis is fitted. These radiographs form the baseline against which any future loss of bone can be measured. Maintenance care is an important aspect of caring for patients who have received implant-retained restorations. The maintenance care regime should include regular checking of the patient's oral hygiene and the condition of the gingival tissues around the implant-retained prostheses. This regular follow-up is crucial as it enables any complications to be picked up early. For screw-retained prostheses, the prosthesis should be removed and checked at the recall appointment. The gingival tissues are assessed using bleeding and probing into the gingival sulcus. The success rates of single unit implant-retained crowns have been reported to be as high as 95% and those of multiple units range from 85 to 98% depending on the preoperative situation in the mouth. Patients must take the responsibility for maintaining their prosthesis long term.

Conclusion

The use of dental implants to restore missing teeth is a commonly used technique. A number of different systems are available offering slight advantages over one another. It is crucial that whichever system is used, there is simplicity in the procedure. Although there are a number of implant systems available, the assessment and planning related to the case are the critical determinants of optimal success. It is important to remember that badly planned and placed implant-retained restorations can cause more damage than benefit. The ultimate outcome of dental implants is dependant on close team working between the clinician, nurse and the patient, and hence knowledge of the procedures and techniques is valuable in ensuring the most predictable outcomes. Today consumer-driven demands have pushed the boundaries to an extent where implants are being placed soon after extraction and also loaded immediately after placement, but the soft tissue envelope still remains challenging and will continue to pose difficulties as we get more adventurous with our surgical and prosthetic techniques.

Maintenance 7

Success rates have been calculated for fixtures and prostheses. For fixtures the rates quoted range from 95 to 99% in the mandible and from 85 to 94% in the maxilla. For prosthetic outcomes the rates quoted are slightly less. It is important that success and survival rates are interpreted carefully. A surviving implant is not necessarily a successful implant. To achieve the success rates quoted, the case needs to be carefully planned and assessed. However, to ensure the successful outcome of dental implant treatment regular monitoring and maintenance of the implant-retained prosthesis once it is fitted are essential.

During the course of such treatment complications may arise at any time during the first year after treatment or longer, depending on the individual case. These complications can be categorized as:

- short-term complications, which occur immediately postoperatively or during the course of treatment
- long-term complications, which may manifest themselves after the implant-retained prosthesis has been functioning for many years.

These complications are best managed if they are detected and diagnosed early and appropriate corrective measures are implemented.

Short-term complications

These can be divided into the following:

- post-surgical complications
- integration failure.

Post-surgical complications

These complications occur within a few days of the surgical placement of the implant. It is important that the patient is warned about postoperative swelling, pain and discomfort, bleeding and bruising as well as the feeling of lingering numbness in the operated site, which are normal side effects of the surgical procedure. All these complications are short term and often resolve within the first week. Patients should be reassured and given advice on how to manage these different complications. The use of regular pain killers to alleviate the pain should also be discussed. The swelling could be minimized by the use of ice packs immediate postoperatively and the patient should be reassured that the swelling will dissipate after a couple of days. Bleeding can occur and should be controlled with moderate pressure to the area using gauze packs.

Although infections are not a common complication, these can occur with poor surgical technique or sometimes if the patient is feeling run down. If the pain does not resolve and is worsening after the surgery, and the patient is complaining of a bad taste, it is likely that there has been some infection and appropriate antibiotics will need to be prescribed.

Partial numbness can be experienced, especially in the mandible, and occurs as a result of either temporary fluid pressure on the nerve or trauma to the nerve during surgery. This is usually short lived, but in some cases it can extend over longer periods of time, depending on the procedure undertaken at surgery.

Integration failure

Although rare, failure of the implant to integrate into the jaw does occur and this can be traumatizing for the both patient and the operator. A failed implant does not normally cause any discomfort, but sometimes localized inflammation around the gingivae is noted on palpation. Although the cause of failure often remains unknown, there are several factors that may contribute to it. The most common is disturbance of the fixture during the initial healing period. To minimize this risk, removable dentures should not be worn in the immediate healing period. Smoking also affects the local blood supply and has been associated with a higher risk of failure (see Fig. 7.1). Other factors that may be contributory to failure are infection in the site of fixture placement and poor surgical technique during the placement, with overheating of the bone. Implants placed in grafted bone sometimes fail to integrate due to poor vascularity (see Fig. 7.2).

Other complications that can occur in the short term are exposure of the bone graft or membrane if augmentation has been used. If these occur then local measures need to be used to ensure that the implanted site does not get infected.

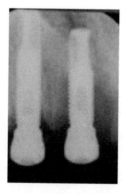

Figure 7.1 Radiograph of a failing implant in a heavy smoker. The radiolucency around the distal implant is evident

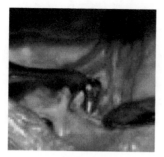

Figure 7.2 Failed fixture placed in bone grafted from the hip. Note the site has poor vascularity

Long-term complications

These complications are usually seen after the implant-retained prosthesis has been functioning for some time. These complications can be grouped as follows:

- soft tissue complications
- poor positioning
- biomechanical failure
- loss of integration.

Soft tissue complications

The most common problem that patients with missing teeth present with is the loss of soft tissue. This usually occurs due to poor extraction technique and poor design of the replacement prosthesis, which impinges on the wound during

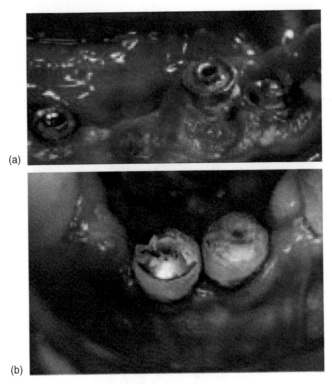

(a)

(b)

Figure 7.3   **(a)** Poor oral hygiene around fixtures, which has caused extensive inflammation of the tissue. Despite this there are no probing depths >3 mm. **(b)** Calculus deposits on healing abutments

healing thus exacerbating bone loss. To minimize any such complications soft tissue factors should be taken into consideration during the planning phases. In patients with poor oral hygiene the presence of plaque and debris around the implants can contribute to localized marginal inflammation of the gingival tissues. This is often referred to as peri-implant mucositis, where only the marginal gingival tissue is affected with no bone loss. The condition reverses itself with a course of oral hygiene instruction and improved cleaning (see Figs 7.3a, b). Implant-retained prostheses that are poorly maintained may also show gingival tissue inflammation with swelling (see Fig. 7.4). Peri-implant mucositis is managed locally with improved oral hygiene and irrigation with chlorhexidine.

Occasionally persistent irritation may cause gingival tissue proliferation. In some instances the inflammation may extend to involve the bone and this is recognized with progressive bone loss. The bone loss is seen as a circumferential defect and normally progresses rapidly (see Loss of integration section). This condition is called peri-implantitis. Management of this condition is by assessing

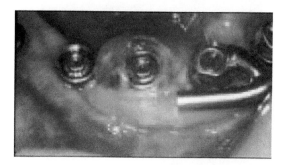

Figure 7.4 Localized inflammation associated with fixtures with no other severe breakdown. This was associated with loose abutment and poor cleaning. This localized inflammation is called peri-implant mucositis

the occlusion, intervening with cleaning after removal of the prosthesis. If the condition does not stabilize surgical intervention may be necessary (see Figs 7.5a–c).

Poor positioning of the implant

The positioning of implants is the key to successful outcome and requires careful planning both prior to and during the surgical placement. Implants placed in poor positions are difficult to restore and can cause problems with biomechanical failure or on occasion implant failure due to overload. Badly placed implants will also cause aesthetic failures (see Fig. 7.6). Additionally, if adequate space is not allowed between the implants and teeth, the space required for cleaning will be compromised, contributing to the soft tissue inflammation discussed above.

Biomechanical failure

These failures include problems with the prosthetic screw loosening and the breakage of implant components. Screw loosening is the most common problem reported, especially with single crowns. To minimize this problem it is crucial that the screw is torqued to the required level using the appropriate torque-controlling devices. This problem was more common with external hex implants and is not seen that frequently with internal connections. If the prosthetic screw repeatedly loosens, then there may be some occlusal overload that needs to be checked. The abutment screw can also loosen and this becomes more difficult in the cement-retained prosthesis where the crown may need to be cut off to access the screw hole. Fig. 7.7 shows a fractured abutment screw in a patient with bruxism. This same patient presented with signs of peri-implantitis and ultimately the implants were lost.

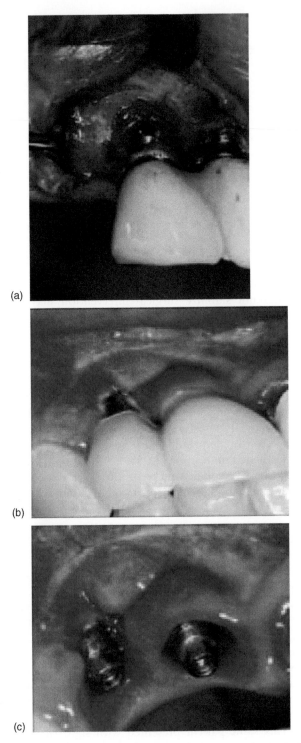

Figure 7.5 (a) Circumferential bone loss, which is typical of a peri-implantitis lesion. (b, c) Inflammation around implants with poor access for cleaning. This caused recurrent abscesses with bone loss

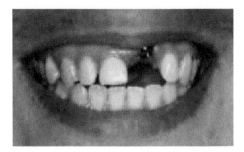

Figure 7.6   Fixture placed in a poor position in a patient with a high smile line, compromising the appearance

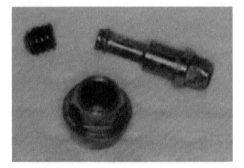

Figure 7.7   Fractured abutment screw in a patient who was grinding his teeth

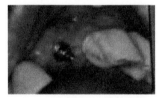

Figure 7.8   Fracture provisional bridge in a patient with unfavourable occlusion

The other common failure seen is fracture of the prosthesis. If this occurs then the material used to construct the prosthesis needs to be assessed and checked. Occasionally breakage of the implant and/or abutment can also occur. This is most likely due to either poor positioning of the implant and/or overload as a result of poor planning (see Fig. 7.8).

Iatrogenic failures of the screws can occur and care must be taken during the removal and placement of the screws into the prosthesis.

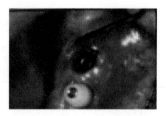

Figure 7.9   Probing around an implant-retained prosthesis to ensure health

Loss of integration

Well-functioning implants can undergo extensive bone loss over a period of time. Although the cause of this remains unclear, two theories have been postulated. One is that of excessive load on the implant during chewing and grinding, for example parafunctional activity, and the second is the presence of bacterial infection at the peri-implant mucosa causing an inflammatory reaction similar to that seen in periodontitis patients. The bone loss seen is usually catastrophic due to the lack of a periodontal ligament. This type of severe bone loss, when seen around implants, is called peri-implantitis. If this type of bone loss is occurring it is important that the occlusion is checked and adjusted and a nightguard provided. Clinical monitoring and assessing of the gingival tissues and the pockets around the implants as well as radiographs are used to detect such changes (Fig. 7.9). Additionally, if oral hygiene is compromised then this needs to be improved and local irrigation with chlorhexidine may be required. On occasion surgical access to clean the area is considered. Implants that have suffered a peri-implantitis reaction can be salvaged, but it is important that the lesion is detected early.

Follow-up and maintenance care

To ensure that complications related to implant-retained prostheses are kept to a minimum, regular maintenance care and follow-up are crucial. Problems that are detected early have a higher chance of being managed whereas those that are detected late may lead to loss of the implant and the retained prosthesis. Oral hygiene should be performed on a regular basis with the appropriate cleaning tools to access the teeth. The gingival tissues around the implant should be monitored regularly using plastic probes for any early signs of inflammation and bleeding. The use of abrasive powders and brushes should be avoided as this will scratch the surface of the titanium, creating a plaque trap. The intervals for recall and follow-up should be customized to individual patients although it is important that radiographic assessments are undertaken on a regular basis, especially in the presence of persistent inflammation. With the two-stage systems more bone loss is seen around the neck of the implant (up to 1 mm) in the first year, whereas with the Straumann system this is seen over 2 years.

A typical maintenance visit for a patient restored with dental implants should comprise:

- an assessment of any concerns the patient may have
- an update of the patient's medical history
- a clinical assessment, which should include the following:
    - an oral hygiene assessment, which should include an assessment of the patient's ability to clean under the prosthesis, especially around the implant abutments
    - looking for the presence of bleeding or suppuration around the implants
    - checking for the presence of probing depths, which are usually assessed against the baseline records taken at the end of the active treatment (a standardized plastic probe is used to avoid scratching the implant-retained surface)
    - an assessment of the occlusal surfaces of the teeth and any abnormal signs of wear (if necessary screw-retained prosthesis can be removed and checked)
- radiographic assessment.

If any hard deposits or calculus are noted these should be removed using the appropriate instruments, taking care not to damage the implant abutments. Oral hygiene, if inadequate, should be improved and the patient reinstructed in how to access the difficult areas. The use of chlorhexidine can be recommended, but this should only be advised during periods of acute problems and should not be recommended for long-term use. On average a maintenance visit can last from 30 to 45 minutes if undertaken properly.

The successful outcome of implant treatment is dependant on a combination of factors, including good and careful treatment planning at the outset, proper placement of the implants in the correct position in reference to the intended prosthetic position and the maintenance of the prosthesis afterwards by the patient. Success rates vary from 90 to 95% across all the published studies, but these rates will not be achieved if a careful sequence of planning and postoperative care and follow-up is not initiated. Implantology is a growing and expanding field and successful outcomes within this field are dependant on close and interactive team working, with the team comprising the clinician, the patient and the dental nurses, including the receptionists. The nurses are the most important team members as they will be expected to set the procedure up, and also reassure patients as they often feel more able to openly express their fears to the nursing team than to the clinician.

The dental nurse's role in implantology

8

It is said that for implants to be a success all of the dental team need to be trained (Hobkirk et al. 2003). There are various providers of training for the dental team in this area, including manufacturers of implant systems, dental hospitals and private companies. Training for dental nurses usually comprises 1- or 2-day courses, either in conjunction with clinicians or specifically for dental nurses. Whatever course you choose, remember that as part of the dental team the dental nurse's role is vital to the success of implant procedures.

This chapter will endeavour to give guidelines on the role of the dental nurse during an implant restoration, from a simple single tooth restoration to a full-mouth reconstruction.

The role of the dental nurse in implantology can be broken down into the following stages:

- the initial visit
- the planning stage
- the preparation stage
- the surgery stage
- the post-surgical procedure (postoperative care)
- the second-stage surgery (if part of the treatment plan)
- the abutment fit and the impression stage
- the fit stage
- the review stage.

The initial visit

When patients attend the dental surgery, the suggestion of implants could simply be an outcome of a routine dental check-up, as a treatment option. Some patients may already have implants in mind as it is a treatment option that patients are becoming more familiar with. Whatever the reason for a patient having implant treatment, the dental nurse's role at this initial visit will be to:

- ensure the medical history is taken
- ensure the dental chart is correct, showing the teeth present, the restorative treatment required, the gingival condition and previous dental treatment
- develop radiographs – full-mouth periapicals to dentopantomograms (to assess the feasibility of implant placement)
- mix alginate for study models (for treatment planning to take place)
- assist with the face bow (so the study models can be articulated)
- provide the relevant literature on implant treatment
- support and reassure the patient during the visit
- arrange for the patient's next visit (allowing time for the clinician to plan the treatment).

Instruments

- Mouth mirror
- Straight probe no 6
- CPITN probe
- Periodontal pocket measuring probe, for example UNC15
- College tweezers
- Furcation probe, for example Nabers
- Gauze and cotton wool rolls
- Electric pulp tester
- Personal protection equipment for the patient, clinician and dental nurse, for example safety glasses, bib, mouthwash.

The planning stage

Before the initial visit the clinician will have looked at the evidence and made a preliminary treatment plan. At this visit the treatment plan and what could be achieved will be discussed with the patient.

It is important to listen to the proposed treatment plan as it will allow you to clarify the proposal should the patient want additional information. Remember, part of the dental nurse's role is to provide support and act as a chaperone to the clinician.

At this visit, a diagnostic wax-up of the missing teeth may be necessary, allowing the patient to see the long-term outcome of the treatment. Further special radiographs may also be required, as described in Chapter 6. These radiographs assist the clinician in deciding how good the surrounding alveolar bone is. These radiographs are specialized therefore an appointment for this may have to be arranged. The diagnostic wax-up may also be used to construct a surgical stent.

During this visit the clinician may take an impression for a surgical stent. 'Surgical stents are used to assist in the placement of the dental implant' (Hobkirk et al. 2003).

It may be the responsibility of the dental nurse to arrange for the relevant components to be available. There must always be a stock of the required length of implants. Implant manufacturers have different policies on ordering. For example, some companies allow items purchased to be returned if not required. Both the dental nurse and the clinician need to discuss how much stock is acceptable. Remember, implant components are expensive. When a clinician has decided on what is needed, ensure that these components and disposables are available (see prepping the surgery).

Edentulous patients may require dentures to be made before implant surgery takes place. The role of the dental nurse is the same as when providing a patient with a new denture. Some patients may have a single tooth extracted and a partial denture fitted before the surgery takes place, whereas other patients may have the tooth extracted on the day of surgery and an implant fitted straight away.

Simple replacement of a single tooth

Preoperative preparation for the surgical procedure

Depending on the system used, the drill kits can either be single or multiple use. In the former, the drills are discarded after use. Multiple use drills will need the number of used episodes to be documented. Once the recommended use has been reached, these are discarded. Remember to always have a spare set available.

Implant components – fixtures

It is ideal to have a selection of fixtures either side of the size planned as clinicians can change their minds once the procedure has begun. As previously discussed, many implant manufacturers allow an exchange policy because of the high cost of components. Discuss with the manufacturer the policy that applies to the system you use, not forgetting that the corresponding healing abutments may need to be ordered if necessary.

Order a **surgical drape kit**, which comes in various styles but usually contains:

- sterile gowns ×3
- theatre caps ×3

- patient drape
- sterile bench and bracket table covers
- sterile bag for the drill equipment
- gauze
- aspiration tip and tube
- sterile light handle covers
- sterile aspiration tubing.

If you do not order a designed drape kit, items can be purchased separately. Ensure you have in stock:

- sterile gloves ×3
- face mask/visor
- patient safety glasses (which should be soaked in antiseptic)
- sterile surgical blades usually no. 11/12/15
- vicyrl sutures
- bone trap
- saline bag – 500 ml IV
- local anaesthetic
- needle
- chlorhexidene scrub solution
- needle guard
- topical anaesthetic
- chlorhexidene.

Ensure that the surgical stent has been returned from the laboratory. Soak the stent in dilute hydrochloric acid for 10 minutes, rinse and place in a bowl of chlorhexidine mouthwash.

Preparation for the surgical procedure – surgical placement of the implant fixture

When preparing a dental surgery for implant placement, it is said that asepsis can hold the key to the long-term success of an implant, 'The importance of asepsis in the long-term success of implant procedures cannot be over emphasized' (Garg et al., 2005). It is therefore important that the definitions of asepsis and antisepsis are understood.

Asepsis is the absence of living pathogenic organisms. The procedure used to reduce the risk of bacterial contamination involves:

- the use of sterile instruments
- the use of the no-glove touch technique.

Antisepsis is the removal of transient micro-organisms from the skin and a reduction in the resident flora.

When preparing the dental surgery using asepsis technique ideally there should be two dental nurses, each with a different role. Dental nurse 1 takes the role of the **circulatory** or **non sterile** dental nurse. Dental nurse 2 takes the role of the **sterile** or **scrub** dental nurse. Each dental nurse has a specific duty. Sometimes one dental nurse has to perform both roles. With organization this can be achieved.

General rules of asepsis

- The circulatory (non-sterile) dental nurse should never reach over the sterile area.
- The circulatory (non-sterile) dental nurse and objects should remain at least 30 cm (1 ft) away form all sterile areas.
- The scrub (sterile) dental nurse should only handle sterile items.
- The scrub (sterile) dental nurse is considered sterile on the front only, from the shoulders to the waist.
- If there is any doubt about the sterility of an object or area, it is considered to be non sterile.
- All items in the sterile field must be sterilized according to approved methods (Central Sterile Supply Department) or through a sterilizer with a vacuum drying cycle.

The role of the circulatory dental nurse

- Remove all unnecessary items (such as plants, cups and personal items) from the surgery. Anything not being used for the procedure should be removed.
- Wipe down all horizontal surfaces with an alcohol-based disinfectant cloth, including lights, equipment stands and chair.
- Ideally the walls of the surgery should be wiped with an antiseptic up to 1.21 m (48 in) from the floor.
- The floor should also be cleaned. This can be arranged by ensuring the cleaner has thoroughly mopped and disinfected the floor area prior to the surgical session.
- Gather all necessary supplies.

Pre-operative preparation

Gather all essential items. Always use a checklist to ensure all items are present:

- sterile instruments (surgical kit)
- local anesthetic tray – dental mirror, straight probe, periodontal probe college tweezers, local anaesthetic syringe, needle, cartridges of local anesthetic, topical anaesthetic paste, re-sheathing device, chlorhexidine mouthwash and timer
- materials – additional local anaesthetic cartridges, saline, chlorhexidine mouthwash
- disposables – sterile gowns, sterile needles, sterile scalpel blades, etc.

- implant machinery
- components – drills and fixtures
- a portable suction unit (preferred but not essential)
- a radiographic viewer with the appropriate radiographs displayed
- graft materials.

Basic surgical instruments (all items prepared/autoclaved)

A set of instruments should ideally be purchased for basic surgical procedures Remember, instruments are only deemed sterilized when bagged, and if the sterilizer has a drying vacuum cycle and instruments come out dry on completion of the process. If the sterilizer does not have a drying vacuum cycle and the instruments come out wet, you will be unable to use the bagged system. The instruments should be laid on a tray without touching, placed in the cycle, allowed to cool and taken from the non-vacuumed sterilizer straight to a sterile surface.

The basic instruments required are:

- mirror
- probe no. 6
- college tweezers
- periodontal pocket measuring probe
- scalpel ×2
- periosteal elevator
- tissue forceps
- suture scissors
- needle holders
- retractor
- syringe
- bone ronguers
- artery forceps
- curettes.

Implant equipment

- Drilling unit and motor assembled with a handpiece.
- Disposable hose set for irrigation equipment with a saline infusion bag (500 ml).
- Implant components – as stated before it is ideal to have a selection of fixtures either side of the size planned.
- Healing abutments or similar if the procedure is single stage.
- Bone trap.
- The surgical stent, which should be soaked in chlorhexidine (1 h minimum).
- Additional equipment.
- Special kits for grafting.

Surgical scrub

Step 1
Remove all jewellery on hands and wrists.

Step 2
Adjust the water to a warm temperature and wet hands and forearms thoroughly.

Step 3
Clean under each fingernail with a stick or brush. It is important for all surgical staff to keep their fingernails short.

Step 4
Holding hands up above the level of elbow, apply the antiseptic. Using a circular motion, begin at the fingertips of one hand and lather and wash between the fingers, continuing from fingertip to elbow. Repeat this for the second hand and arm. Continue washing in this way for 3–5 minutes.

Step 5
Rinse each arm separately, fingertips first, holding hands above level of elbow.

Step 6
Using a sterile towel, dry arms – from fingertips to elbow – using a different side of the towel on each arm.

Step 7
Keep hands above the level of waist and do not touch anything before putting on sterile surgical gloves.

Gowning and gloving

- After scrubbing the hands the sterile dental nurse should put on the sterile gloves and gown.
- The sterile dental nurse will set up the sterile work area with the aid of the non-sterile circulating dental nurse.
- All personnel should wear hats and masks whilst setting up the surgery.

Putting on sterile gown and gloves

- Ask the circulating dental nurse to open the packages.
- After scrubbing, the sterile dental nurse should dry hands from the fingers to the elbows using sterile towels.
- Packages such as bone traps, grafting materials and implant fixtures should only be opened during the surgery when the clinician is ready for them.

Gowning

The scrub dental nurse should take hold of the gown, which is folded with the inside facing outwards, placing hands in the sleeves and opening the gown.

Figs 8.1a, b, c and d show the gowning technique.

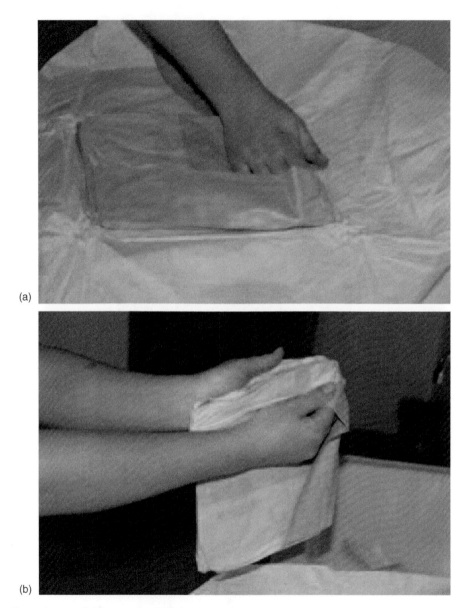

(a)

(b)

Figure 8.1   (a–d) The gowning technique

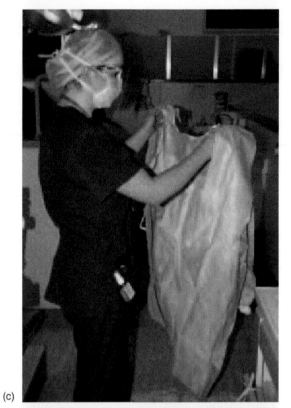

(c)

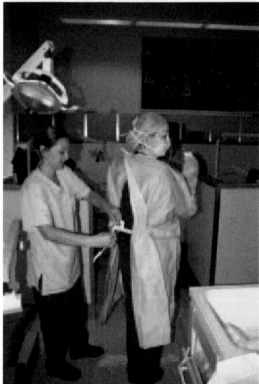

(d)

Figure 8.1 *Continued*

As the scrub dental nurse places the arms in the sleeves, the circulating dental nurse should take hold of the inside of the gown from behind, pull it on and lace the ties at the back. The final tie of the gowning is completed after the gloving procedure.

Gloving

- The circulating dental nurse opens the package containing gloves.
- Taking the inner package, the sterile dental nurse opens it and grasps the folded opening of one glove and places the other hand on it. The fold should not be unrolled.

Figs 8.2a and b show the gloving technique.

- With the gloved hand the scrub dental nurse grasps the fold of the other glove and places it on the hand without touching the outside of either glove.
- The scrub dental nurse should then roll the folded edges of the gloves back over the sleeve opening of the gown.

Gowning

- The scrub dental nurse may now wrap the belt of the gown around and tie it with the assistance of the circulating dental nurse.
- The scrub dental nurse takes the tag and hands the white part to the circulating dental nurse.
- The scrub dental nurse then rotates and pulls away from the circulating dental nurse until the belt can be tied.

Preparing the surgery

- The surgical drape kit is placed on the bracket table and should be opened by the circulating dental nurse so that the outer drape completely covers the bracket table.
- The circulating dental nurse then opens the bags containing the sterile equipment. The scrub dental nurse places the instruments on the bracket table and organizes the instrument drapes.

Bracket table cover

- The bracket table is covered completely
- The scrub dental nurse opens the cover, places hands inside and lifts the cover over the bracket table.
- The circulating dental nurse takes the corners and pulls them over the bracket table.

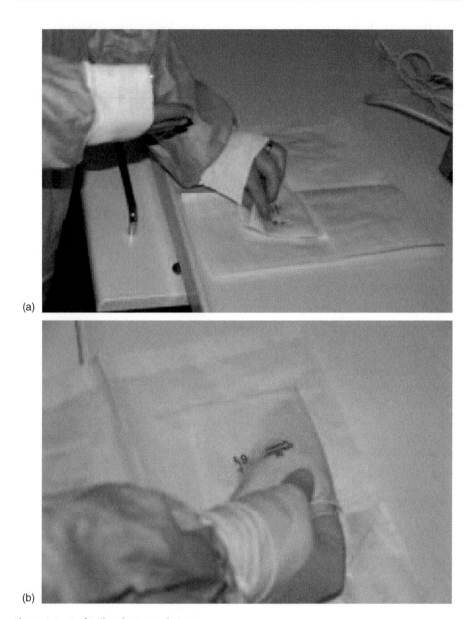

(a)

(b)

Figure 8.2　(a, b) The gloving technique

The drilling equipment and motors

- Both the controller set and drilling equipment should be covered with sterile drapes. The drilling equipment can be placed in a sterile bag provided in the drape kit or covered with a sterile sheet.
- The drilling equipment should be checked, activated and left on stand-by.
- Cables, dental motors and the irrigation bag are connected by the circulating dental nurse and covered with relevant sterile tubing covers.

- The scrub dental nurse places a cover over the cables and dental motor. The circulator dental nurse pulls down the tubing, only touching the fold.

Aspiration system

Connect the aspiration system using suction tubing provided (ideally two aspirator tips should be available so both dental nurses can aspirate during the procedure):

- one aspirator tip to aspirate any saliva and saline from the oral cavity and in particular the back of the throat.
- one aspirator tip to connect to a bone trap as the clinician may wish to collect bone during the site preparation to use for augmentation later. Remember, aspirating with a bone trap means the bone collected should not be contaminated with saliva and hence must not be used to aspirate saliva.

Completion of surgery preparation

- Make sure all areas are covered with sterile drapes until needed.
- Don't forget to prepare a local tray and basic instruments for when the patient first sits in the chair, ideally this should be done elsewhere.
- If the dentist has a surgical stent, bathe the stent in chlorhexidene.

The dental nurse's role during surgery

Preoperative care of the patient

Usually the sterile dental nurse begins prepping the patient whilst the circulatory dental nurse aids the clinician with gowning, and then prepares to become the aspiration dental nurse when the clinician begins the procedure. The sterile dental nurse will become the component nurse during the surgical procedure.

Duties of the circulatory dental nurse:

- Meet and greet the patient.
- Ensure that the patient has eaten before the treatment, and if not then give a glucose drink.
- Check any changes in medical history.
- Make sure the clinician goes through the treatment plan and the patient knows what is going to happen.
- Make sure the consent form is signed.
- When the patient sits in the chair ask the patient to rinse with chlorhexidine mouthwash for 1 minute (use a timer so the patient completes the 1 minute rinse).
- Before the local anaesthetic is given place the theatre cap on the patient.
- Lipstick should be removed.

■ Patients may be given antibiotic cover of 3 g of amoxicillin or 600 mg of clindamycin, depending on the clinician and the patient's previous medical history.

Duties of the sterile nurse

■ When the procedure is about to begin and the patient is draped, wipe the soft tissues with chlorhexidene, stroking away from the oral cavity, using sterile gauze and a pair of artery forceps.

The surgical procedure

The aspiration dental nurse stays on site, keeping the surgical field clear from blood. This dental nurse may also retract the tissues and irrigate the drill if the system does not have internal irrigation.

The component dental nurse will pass dental instruments and load the handpiece with the relevant drills and components. This is where specialist implant training for the relevant system will aid support and knowledge.

As a tip to keep on track with the procedure, always tell the clinician what drill or component you are passing to them. This prevents confusion. Most companies also have simple diagrams of drill sequences that you can laminate and display on the wall. Remember to place all drills back into relevant place so they do not get lost. Remember to rinse the bur in saline as bone can also be collected in this way.

When the clinician has requested the implant, the circulatory nurse opens the packaging, and drops the 'sterile' internal package onto the drape. The component dental nurse will then pick the implant fixture without touching it. Any contact with the implant surface is likely to cause loss of osseointegration.

During the drilling of the bone the speed of the motor is usually set between 800–1000 rpm depending on the system. The implant insertion/placement torque is usually at 25–35 NCM, depending on the bone quality. Therefore remember to adjust the speed of the motor as the implants are being placed.

The aspirating dental nurse must allow the blood to flow as the clinician places the implant; it is always tempting to clear the areas to improve visibility. At this stage refrain from doing so as it allows the socket to have a good supply of blood for ossteointegration to take place.

Once the implant is in place the component dental nurse must make sure that the information on the packaging of the implant is recorded, both in the patient's notes and on a record card for future reference. Implant manufacturers will require as much information as possible regarding the implant placed should it fail.

Following placement of the implant, depending on the technique used, a cover screw will be put in place and the site sutured or a healing abutment put in place. Whatever the procedure, sutures need to be provided and following closure postoperative instruction should be given by the aspirating dental nurse whilst the component dental nurse begins the procedure of clearing away. It is important that the dental nurse remembers to clean the drills immedialely after use.

Postoperative care of the patient

Postoperative advice should be given to the patient by the dental nurse:

- Warn the patient there may be swelling and bruising.
- Use a pressure pack or ice pack to reduce the swelling.
- Pain control – an analgesic may be prescribed; patients are advised to take what they usually take for a headache.
- If a patient is prescribed antibiotics they should complete the course.
- Some patients are prescribed nasal drops, especially if they have had implants placed close to the sinuses. The nasal drops will dry the nose so patients will not have to blow their noses.
- Haemostasis – sterile gauze is provided should bleeding occur.
- Rinsing – saline solution or chlorhexidine mouthwash should be recommended.
- Instructions on keeping the area clean are given.
- An appointment must be given for suture removal.
- Give the patient a contact telephone number for emergencies.
- Some patients may not be allowed to wear their denture at first because of the incision placement.
- If a patient is allowed to wear their denture it should be kept in overnight for the first night.

Cleaning and sterilizing of instruments

Cleaning procedure:

- Sharps should be removed and disposed of (by clinician).
- Surgical instruments should be placed in an ultrasonic bath with general purpose cleaner for 12 minutes, rinsed, scrubbed and dried ready for sterilization.
- Depending on single use or multiple use, the drills may need frequent changing depending on bone density.
- Make a note of the drills discarded so they can be replaced and reordered.
- The drills need careful cleaning with a small toothbrush after use.
- The hand-held screwdrivers, manual torque wrenches and bone mills need to be dismantled before sterilizing and reassembled at use. This depends on the implant system being used. If in doubt contact the manufacturer of the system or look in the catalogue for guidance.
- Components such as direction indicators need to be threaded with floss for safety during use in the mouth. Do not thread with waxed floss as it becomes brittle after the sterilization process.

- When ultrasonic cleaning the drills and loose components, place them in a Pyrex beaker for safety. They are small and can easily be lost.
- Handpieces will need running through, cleaning, dismantling and oiling before sterilization.

Decontamination of the dental surgery and aspiration system

- Clear away all instruments and equipment.
- Decontaminate the dental surgery in the usual way.
- Clean the filter on the aspirator.
- Run the suction unit through with an appropriate disinfectant.
- Re-set the unit for next the patient.
- Have a well earned coffee/tea!

When assisting for the first time with the placement of an implant, an implant regional representative will often, if contacted, come along and give support. Remember to plan and discuss with the clinician the needs of the practice then things should run smoothly because the whole team will know what to expect.

Review appointment

One week following the surgery, the patient will have the sutures removed and a postoperative check. The dental nurse may be required to assist with the suture removal.

Instruments

- Mirror
- Straight probe
- College tweezers
- Suture scissors
- Chlorhexidine mouthwash
- Sterile gauze
- Personal protection equipment
- Postsurgical toothbrush (soft)
- Hand mirror

The dental nurse may be asked to provide oral hygiene instruction.

Second-stage surgery

If a two-stage surgical approach has been organized in the treatment plan, the following protocol is used. Aseptic technique is again important. The area will be opened with a tissue punch or a routine flap will be raised. A basic surgical kit will therefore be required with local anaesthetic.

Aspiration will aid vision for the clinician. Once the implant has been located the clinician may require a bone mill to remove bone that may have grown over the implant cover screw. Bone mills need to be assembled to the manufacturer's instruction. Sterile dental floss should be attached for safety.

Once the cover screw has been removed, the healing abutment will be placed and the area re-sutured so healing can take place.

In the preplanning for this procedure, the dental nurse needs to order the components required for this stage, usually the healing abutments. The dental nurse needs to ensure that the clinician decides on the required components so they can be ordered and received before the patient attends. When healing has taken place an appointment will be made for the impressions to be taken.

The prosthodontic stage

Following second-stage surgery and fitting of the healing abutment the prosthodontic stage takes place. The clinical time for the stages can vary from one visit to several visits, depending on the complexity of the individual case.

As impressions for the prosthetic restoration is the next treatment stage, ensure that the relevant impression copings and abutments are available for the patient's visit. Planning and preparation for this stage are just as important as surgery preparation. Discuss with the clinician which type of impression will be taken so that relevant impression copings and abutments can be ordered. The clinician may require a range of sizes of abutments as for implant placement. At this visit the healing abutments will be removed and the abutment and impression copings will be positioned.

The purpose of the implant level impression is to relate the position of the implant platform to other implants, teeth and soft tissue contours. The implant level impression is generally made after second-stage surgery, after a healing abutment has been in place and the gingival cuff has formed (Nobel Biocare 2002).

The clinician has the choice of two impression techniques: the closed-tray technique and the open-tray technique.

Closed-tray technique

The impression copings stay in the mouth attached to the abutment or implant fixture as the impression is taken out. The copings are then removed and reseated into the indentations in the impression. This provides an accurate position for the implants.

Open-tray technique

The impression copings are still connected to the abutments or implant fixtures, but the screws project holding the impression coping first have to be released and then the impression can be removed from the mouth. The copings are securely fixed in the impression once set.

Whatever technique is chosen, the clinician will use an elastomeric impression material. It is vital that standard infection control protocols are followed when mixing the impression material and before the impression is sent to the laboratory. It is usual for light body impression material to be syringed around the impression coping. The heavy body is mixed and loaded in the tray as with a standard crown or bridge impression.

An occlusal registration is taken using a face-bow either at this stage or the next visit. An opposing impression is then taken so that the study model can be articulated for the technician to have a true replica of the occlusion. Inter-occlusal records will also help as implants must not be heavily loaded. Mousse or wax can be used for taking these records. A shade for the crown or bridge will also be taken. During shade taking, remember to adjust the dental light away from the patient to give as much natural light as possible; sometimes this may mean asking the patient to stand by the window. After the impressions protective silicone caps are replaced onto the abutments before the patient leaves or healing caps replaced onto the implant fixtures. Some patients are happy to stay like this until the permanent crown or bridge can be fitted. Temporary crowns or bridges can be made. If this is the case the temporary crown or bridge will be fitted using a temporary material. If temporary dentures are being worn then the healing abutment may be replaced so the patient can continue to wear the dentures until the final crown or bridge work is ready.

Instruments and materials required for the impression stage

- Mirror
- Probe
- Periodontal pocket measuring probe (to help select the height of the final abutment)
- College tweezers
- Local anaesthetic (in case of overgrowth of the tissues around the healing abutment)
- Sterile scalpel handle and blade (so adjustment can be done if overgrowth has occurred)
- Hand-held screwdrivers (for removing healing abutment and placing the final abutment)
- Bone mill with dental floss attached as a safety measure (for removing excess bone growth over the fixture if the healing abutment has become loose since second-stage surgery)

- Impression copings for either open-tray or closed-tray technique
- Radiographs (to check copings are down or if there is a problem with the implant)
- Disposable impressions trays (upper and lower with handles)
- Universal adhesive
- Alginate
- Silicone impression material (light and heavy body), guns and tips
- Pink modelling wax for covering open-tray holes (this helps to support the heavy bodied impression material)
- Scissors (for trimming temporary crowns)
- Handpiece – acrylic trimmer, polishing burs
- Temporary crown forms
- Temporary cement for crowns
- Dappens pot (for monomer)
- Spatula and pad
- Shade guide (vita lumin)
- Universal adhesive (to attach material to tray)
- Integrity and gun or trim (to make temporary crowns)
- Articulating paper with Miller forceps ×2 (to check occlusion)
- Face-bow
- Wax
- Ultrasonic bath (to clean healing abutments if being replaced until final work)
- Jaw registration paste

Procedure for a single tooth restoration

Closed-tray impression at abutment level

- Remove healing abutment from implant fixture and place the abutment on the fixture
- Radiographic confirmation of abutment fitting
- Radiographic confirmation of seating of coping
- Final tightening of abutment with torque wrench
- Impression procedure
- Jaw registration
- Shade
- Provide a temporary crown, a protective silicone cap or refit a partial denture following removal of the abutment and replacement of the healing abutment

Procedure for a single tooth restoration using an open-tray impression

- Remove the healing abutment
- Place impression coping directly to the implant

- Radiographic confirmation of abutment fit
- Take impression
- Unscrew the impression coping so the impression can be removed from the mouth
- Replace the healing abutment

This is sent to the laboratory for the abutment and crown to be made. The customized abutment and crown can be made at the same time.

Procedure for multiple restorative case (bridge) (Searson et al. 2005)

This process is similar to that for a single tooth but with more implants.

- Remove any partial dentures or bridges
- Select the abutments (if the impression is abutment leve)
- Remove the healing abutments
- If the patient is wearing a temporary bridge the temporary abutments may already be in place which will need to be removed
- Seat the impression copings either on fixture or abutment
- Take a radiograph to confirm the fit
- Take an impression
- Depending on number of teeth remaining, either jaw registration and occusal record can be taken at this visit or may need another visit
- Jaw registration sent to the laboratory
- Occlusal record sent to the laboratory
- Re-cement the temporary bridge or replace the partial denture/bridge
- Try and check the bridge on the patient's return visit
- Metal try-in (if the bridge is extensive this is advisable so the thickness of the porcelain or acrylic can be assessed)
- Make final placement of restoration

Try-in and fit stage of an implant prosthesis

At the try-in stage check the following:

- the contours and shape of the restoration
- the occlusion
- if any adjustments are required to the crown or bridge
- that the abutment and crown are seated correctly
- the patient's opinion

On confirmation of fit and appearance the laboratory will finish the restoration and add porcelain, with the staining and glazing. The crown or bridge will then be ready for fitting at the next visit.

Fitting of prostheses

Implant crowns or bridges can be screw or cement retained. There are three types of screw-retained prosthesis:

- screw retained direct to the implant body
- screw retained direct to an abutment
- screw retained with a lateral screw on custom-made abutments.

Cement-retained prostheses may be placed on pre-manufactured or custom-made abutments.

Once the final adjustment has been made the crown or bridge is cemented using a luting cement. It is essential that the crown or bridge is not over-filled with cement. Dental floss and damp gauze can be used to remove excess cement. Good aspiration may also be required.

If the prosthesis is screw retained, gold or titanium prosthetic screws are used to connect the restorative to the abutment. You will need to ensure that the appropriate implant screwdrivers are available. Gauze is often placed in the oral cavity to prevent inhalation of the small screw should it be dropped. The screw head should be protected and sealed with an impression material that is easy to remove (Hobkirk et al. 2003) (Nobel Biocare 2002).

Postoperative instruction

Following the fitting of the crown or bridge postoperative care should be given. Good oral hygiene is essential to ensure the stability of the restoration. The importance of the patient's home maintenance cannot be over-emphasized. Toothbrushing techniques should be reinforced, and flossing and interspace cleaning checked. A review appointment should be arranged in case of any problems.

A follow-up routine scaling and polishing appointment may be arranged as a preventive treatment. The scalers and curettes used for this procedure need to be titanium friendly, and plastic or gold tipped.

Procedure for an edentulous patient with full over-dentures

Dentures can be retained using either a ball attachment or a bar-retained on the implant. These dentures are called over-dentures:

- **A ball attachment denture** is a tissue supported conventional over-denture retained by abutments that are connected directly into the implants.
- **A bar-retained over-denture** is a conventional acrylic denture retained by clips which fit onto a bar.

The denture is usually tissue supported and implant supported. Intra-oral considerations and manual dexterity will determine the type of over-denture (Nobel Biocare 2002) to be used.

The prosthetic stages for implant-retained over-dentures are very similar to routine full/full denture construction. On removal of the healing abutments the fixture/abutment head is sealed using a silicone cap. A primary impression is taken to enable the position of the implants to be recorded. The impression can be taken in a stock tray using impression compound or silicone putty with a wash. This should provide a detailed impression so the special trays can be made. If the prosthesis is to be fixed, a special tray can be constructed with holes added so that an open-tray technique can be used. The abutments are connected at the next visit and secondary impressions taken in elastomeric impression material.

A jaw registration is taken at the next visit with a wax rim on an acrylic base. Once the jaw registration has been taken, teeth are selected and a shade is chosen. At the next visit at the try-in, when the denture is set in wax, the aesthetics and occlusion as well as the lip support is checked. The metal framework, if it is a bar retained over-denture, will also be checked as the next appointment for fit. Once the bar is seated passively at the next visit both the wax and metal are tried in together and if all is well the laboratory is instructed to finish. On the final visit the bar and denture are fitted and postoperative care and maintenance are given for both the denture and the implant. If the denture is a 'ball' retained over-denture then the 'bar' try-in stage is omitted and the secondary impression taken at abutment level after the ball abutment is connected.

Postoperative care for dentures and implants

- Dentures should be cleaned following a meal wherever possible and the mouth rinsed.
- Dentures should be left out at night because of reduced saliva flow.
- Cleaning the denture should be done over a basin of water using a soft toothbrush and soap.
- The dentures should be kept in water to prevent them from drying out.
- Clean the abutment fixtures using an interspace toothbrush, toothpaste and floss.
- If a patient should experience any problems they should contact the surgery for advice or ask for help at a follow-up appointment.

These are guidelines to assist the dental nurse during the process of implant restorative treatment. However, as with any dental treatment techniques may vary as clinicians have their own preferences and adaptations to a treatment plan. Hopefully the guidelines will aid understanding and enhance the nurse's ability to pre-empt and anticipate the needs of the patient and clinician. Be prepared to adapt these techniques as treatments for dental implants develop.

Glossary

Abutment: Usually made of metal or ceramic. Connects to the top of the fixture and extends through the gingivae to the oral cavity. It may consist of one or more components. There are different types of abutment designed for specific tasks.

Abutment replica: A copy of the abutment which is used to construct the prosthesis.

Abutment screw: The screw that secures the abutment to the fixture.

Allogenic bone: Bone tissue from the same type of individuals.

Alloplastic material: Synthetically derived material that does not have a human or animal source. Materials such as bioactive glass, calcium phosphate, hydroxyapatite and calcium sulphate fall into this category.

Antirotation: A feature that prevents the rotation of two joint components, for example abutment to fixture.

Augmentation: A procedure used to try and re-establish the required bone width and height to facilitate fixture placement. This is sometimes called bone grafting.

Autogenous bone: Bone obtained from the same individual used for bone augmentation. The site can be from within the mouth or outside the mouth.

Barrier: Also called a membrane, this is used in guided bone regeneration to help exclude unwanted cells from growing into the defect. The membranes can be non-resorbable or resorbable.

Biocompatible: Ability of a material to function without a negative response from the host (immune response) in a specific application.

CAD/CAM: Computer-aided design/computer-assisted manufacture.

Cement retained: The used of a cement to retain the prosthesis to the abutment.

Computerized tomogram (CT) scan: An X-ray machine that can deliver sectional X-ray pictures in small intervals in three different dimensions (panoramic, cross-sectional, and axial).

Connective tissue graft: Graft of the underlying connective tissue used to increase the thickness of the gum tissue.

Countersink: The last drill in the sequence of drills used to flare the coronal aspect of the site such that the fixture can be placed just below the crest of the bone. This is also called the profile drill or counterbore.

Delayed placement: Fixtures are placed into the socket at least 6–8 weeks after the extraction.

Dental implant: A device placed within, or on, the bone of the jaws (maxilla or mandible) to provide support for a prosthetic reconstruction, which could be a single tooth, multiple teeth or all the teeth (for example, a denture).

Diagnostic wax-up: A replica of the intended position of the teeth and/or gingivae tissue in wax on a stone cast of the patient's mouth. This is usually undertaken in the laboratory. It is used to assess the feasibility of a treatment plan, and tp construct the radiographic guide and the surgical guide.

Duralay jig: Also know as the locating jig. A laboratory fabricated device used to maintain the correct positional relationship of a component when transferring it from the cast to the mouth.

External hex: The type of connection which sits on top of the fixture and connects the abutments.

Fixed prosthesis: A prosthesis which replaces missing teeth and is fixed onto the implants. It cannot be removed by the patient. This is also called a bridge.

Fixture: This is also called the screw or implant and is the part of the implant that is surgically placed into the jaw bone to osseointegrate.

Fixture (implant) analogue: A copy of the implant placed in the mouth that is used by the laboratory.

Free gingival graft: Soft tissue graft of the keratinized gingival tissue used to increase the width of attached (keratinized) gingival tissue.

Guide drill: Round-shaped drill used to mark the site of the osteotomy by making an entry into the cortical bone. This is usually the first drill used.

Guided bone regeneration: Procedure used to help rebuild the bone by using a technique which selectively allows bone cells only to grow into the defect.

Healing abutment: This is used after the surgical phase to guide the gingival tissues to heal into a specific way to enhance aesthetics. Also called healing caps or gingivae formers. They can be made of metal or reinforced plastic.

Immediate loading: When the fixtures are placed and restored at the same time as crowns or dentures and the patient can bite and chew on them straightway.

Immediate placement: Fixtures are placed into the socket at the same time as tooth extraction.

Implant-retained prosthesis: A restoration retained and supported by dental implants.

Impression coping: A device that registers the position of a dental implant or abutment in an impression.

Internal hex: This connection is within the body of the fixture and connects the abutment.

Keratinized gingivae: Part of the oral mucosa covering the gingivae and hard palate and consisting of the free and attached gingivae.

Maintenance care: A structured regime of monitoring and assessment to ensure that the implant-retained prosthesis remains healthy.

One-stage surgery: The fixture is placed into the jaw bone and connected to the mouth with a healing abutment. A prosthetic abutment can also be connected instead of the healing abutment.

Osseointegration: A process whereby clinically asymptomatic and rigid fixation of an alloplastic material is achieved, and maintained, in bone during functional loading.

Peri-implant mucositis: Inflammation of the gingival tissues as a result of poor cleaning which can be resolved with improved cleaning. There is no associated bone loss.

Peri-implantitis: Inflammation of the gingival tissues in conjunction with bone loss. It has been compared to periodontitis.

Position indicator: A device used during the preparation of the fixture site to ascertain the alignment fixture position. Different sizes to match the different drills are used. They are also called alignment pins or guide pins.

Primary stability: Also know as the initial stability, this is the degree of tightness of an implant immediately after placement into the prepared site.

Prosthesis: Also called the restoration, this replaces the teeth and gingivae.

Prosthetic abutments: These are used to retain the crown. They can be preformed or customized to a specific shape.

Prosthetic screw: This is the screw used to secure the crown to the abutment.

Provisional restoration: Temporary restoration placed on the fixtures using temporary abutments.

Radiographic guide: A guide (also called a template) that is made from the diagnostic wax-up that the patient wears when the specialized radiograph is taken. It shows the tooth position in relation to the underlying bone.

Ramus implant: This implant is fixed in the ramus of the mandible, hence its name.

Removable prosthesis: A prosthesis that is retained on the implants and can be removed by the patient. It is also called a denture and normally replaces missing teeth and soft tissue. It can be retained on a bar or on studs.

Retaining screw: A screw used during the construction of the prosthesis to retain it on the cast.

Screw retained: The use of a screw to retain the prosthesis on the abutment.

Screw tap: A device used in the final stages of fixture site preparation, usually in dense bone so that the fixture can be inserted without causing any frictional heat.

Second-stage surgery: A minor surgical procedure to expose the fixture to the mouth.

Sinus augmentation: Procedure undertaken to increase the bone height in the posterior maxilla when there is inadequate bone height to place the fixtures.

Standard placement: Fixtures are placed 6 months after the extraction.

Subperiosteal implants: Implants that lie on top of the jawbone underneath the gingivae tissue but do not penetrate into the jawbone.

Surgical guide: A guide (also called a template) used during surgery to ensure that the fixtures are placed in the correct position in relation to the intended position of the crowns.

Tomograms: Specialized radiographs that are taken to ascertain the bone volume in the patient's mouth.

Torque driver: An instrument used to apply the correct level of tightening (torque) to the screws (abutment or prosthetic). Most companies now offer these as manual devices.

Transosseous implants: Implants that penetrate the whole height of the jaw with one aspect fixed at the lower border or the jaw and the other supporting the teeth projecting through the gingivae. Due to its nature it is mainly used in the anterior part of the mandible.

Two-stage surgery: The fixture is placed in the jaw bone and covered over with the gingival tissue. A small minor procedure is needed to uncover the fixture and connect to the oral cavity.

Xenogenic bone: Bone tissue from a different species, for example bovine (cow), used for grafting.

Appendix

Outline of the clinical protocol for patients undergoing implant treatment

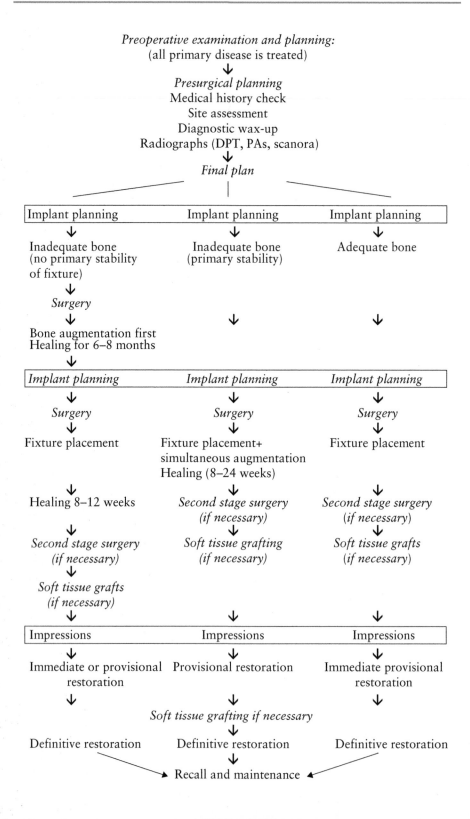

Preoperative examination and planning:
(all primary disease is treated)
↓
Presurgical planning
Medical history check
Site assessment
Diagnostic wax-up
Radiographs (DPT, PAs, scanora)
↓
Final plan

Implant planning	Implant planning	Implant planning
↓	↓	↓
Inadequate bone (no primary stability of fixture)	Inadequate bone (primary stability)	Adequate bone
↓		
Surgery		
↓	↓	↓
Bone augmentation first Healing for 6–8 months		
↓		

Implant planning	*Implant planning*	*Implant planning*
↓	↓	↓
Surgery	*Surgery*	*Surgery*
↓	↓	↓
Fixture placement	Fixture placement+ simultaneous augmentation Healing (8–24 weeks)	Fixture placement
↓	↓	↓
Healing 8–12 weeks	*Second stage surgery (if necessary)*	*Second stage surgery (if necessary)*
↓	↓	↓
Second stage surgery (if necessary)	*Soft tissue grafting (if necessary)*	*Soft tissue grafts (if necessary)*
↓		
Soft tissue grafts (if necessary)		
↓	↓	↓

Impressions	Impressions	Impressions
↓	↓	↓
Immediate or provisional restoration	Provisional restoration	Immediate provisional restoration
↓	↓	↓

Soft tissue grafting if necessary
↓

Definitive restoration	Definitive restoration	Definitive restoration

→ Recall and maintenance ←

Bibliography

Brånemark, P. I., Adell, R., Breine, U., Hansson, B. O., Lindström, J. and Ohlsson, A. 1969 Intra-osseous anchorage of dental prostheses. Part 1: Experimental studies. *Scand J Plast Reconstr Surg* 3 (2), 81–100.

Garg, A. K., Reddi, S. N. and Chacon, G. E. (2005) The importance of asepsis in dental implantology. In: *The Implant Society*, Stradis Healthcare, Georgia. http://www.stradismed.com/resources_article.html.

Hobkirk, J. A., Watson, R. M. and Searson, L. (2003) *Introducing Dental Implants*. Churchill Livingstone/Elsevier, Edinburgh.

Restorative Manual, Nobel Biocare; 2002. (Nobel Biocare, The Grand Union Office Park, Packet Boat Lane, Uxbridge UB8 2GH, UK).

Searson, L., Gough, M. and Hemmings, K. (2005) *Implantology in General Dental Practice*. Quintessential Publishing Co. Ltd, London. http://www.engenderhealth.org/IP/surgical/sum3.html.

Zarb, G. and Albrektsson, T. (1991): Osseointegration: A requiem for this periodontal ligament? The *International Journal of Periodontics & Restorative Dentistry*, 11, 88–91.

Bibliography

Index

Printed and bound by CPI Group (UK) Ltd, Croydon, CR0 4YY

Printed and bound by CPI Group (UK) Ltd, Croydon, CR0 4YY

06/10/2024

14569015-0003